Praise

"While it is about dieting and weight loss as an attempt to try to fit in to a world that demands a certain body shape for women, that is not the entire purpose of this book. *Squeezing Your Size 14 Self into a Size 6 World* is about trying to fit yourself into other people's ideas of what you should be. This book is about breaking free from the molds you are trying to squeeze into just to satisfy others. Throughout the book Carrie Smith provides a gentle coaching method to get you to start breaking free and living a life true to yourself." **Harold McFarland, Readers Preference Reviews**

"Squeezing Your Size 14 Self into a Size 6 World is a must-read for any woman seeking practical solutions for lifelong health, fitness and greater self-acceptance. Smith shares her personal experience and professional expertise as a wellness coach to dispel longstanding misconceptions about diet, body image and fitness. Her advice and guidance on exercise is informed, honest – and 100 percent doable." **Amanda Vogel, MA Human Kinetics, Vice President, FitCity for Women, Vancouver, British Columbia**

"Chapter after chapter, Smith hits the nail on the head. She consistently goes against the quick-fix theories (and rightfully so!) and presents sound, healthy advice that virtually everyone needs to hear. Read, and re-read this book!" **John Acquaviva, PhD, Professor of Exercise Physiology**

"What a lifesaver! This should be required reading for all females throughout their lifespan! As a teacher and coach myself, I can attest to the fact that in order for one to experience true growth, one must learn how to be their own teacher/coach. The 'Coaching Moments' provided in this book allow the reader to become just that: an active participant (self-teacher) in the quest for developing a healthy mind-set about body image. This book is fabulous!" **Michele S. Olson, PhD, FACSM Professor, Exercise Science, Auburn University, Montgomery**

"Carrie Myers Smith exposes every woman's dilemma about squeezing into a size 6 world. She understands how desperate we are to do it, then she sets us straight. Why not exhale, sit down and read what Carrie has to say before you start your next diet? I believe it will make all the difference in achieving the goal of changing your body for the better." **Dr. Deborah Newman, author of** *Loving Your Body*

"Carrie Myers Smith has offered women the ultimate gift through *Squeezing Your Size 14 Self into a Size 6 World.* With a friendly voice of experience, Carrie gives us permission to be who we really are, validation that who and what we are is good, and encouragement with a roadmap to be even better. Using a supportive yet authoritative tone, Myers Smith exposes the truth about self-defeating molds that society forces on us and we force on ourselves, then lights the path to a better way of living." **Victoria L. Freeman, PhD, Health/Fitness Writer & Wellness Coach, Denver, Colorado**

"Finally, a book the focuses on what really matters for women who want to lead healthier and more joyful lives. The Author brings together crucial elements that one must consider when changing a mindset and changing one's life for the better. This is one book that is a must-read for anyone considering a healthy lifestyle change!" **Susan Cantwell, President of The Lifestyle Coaching Institute, author of** *Mind Over Matter,* **Nike® Sponsored Fitness Athlete**

What real women are saying about this book...

"This book is like sitting down and chatting with Carrie—it's very informal and laid back. Before you're finished with this book, you'll be looking at things with a new perspective. I love the way that change is presented as a process (a trip) and moving forward. I am especially impressed by how Carrie overcame anorexia with such insight. It's a powerful book especially for young women today who may by persuaded by media's images of what being 'beautiful' means." **Dara Barth, Colorado**

"*Squeezing Your Size 14 into a Size 6 World* is not only inspiring, but it gives many wonderful and practical ideas, tips, and helps to women at all stages of their lives. Carrie Myers Smith uses her unique sense of humor to be relatable to all of us gals. She is right there with you, coaching you along. What a great opportunity to have your own personal coach with you at all times!" **Linda Kraft, New Hampshire**

"This is an honest look into what it means to be a woman in today's world. Carrie is not afraid to speak the truth about what lies behind our struggles to live a healthy, fulfilling life. She hits the real issues we face, as women, head on with real answers. Get ready to destroy the myth of what we believe to be fitness and embrace what lies beyond the myth . . . a true image of fit." **Julie Saunders, Virginia**

"Carrie Myers Smith has outdone herself with *Squeezing Your Size 14 into a Size 6 World*. Her book has a real-woman approach to fitness and self image in which we can truly identify. I love the way she guides us to set and achieve goals we can actually meet!" **MaryAnn Koopmann, Wisconsin**

"*Squeezing Your Size 14 into a Size 6 World* is a godsend! This book is about a lifestyle and a way of living versus a quick fix. What I appreciate most about this book is the coaching moments that help you reflect and grow. This is a book that can be read time and time again when you need it. So often tools are used once and then put aside, this book is one you will read more than once. It is refreshing to read a book by someone who has gone through the same struggles as I have and is successful. It has given me new inspiration to reach my goals!" **Sara Pattow, Wisconsin**

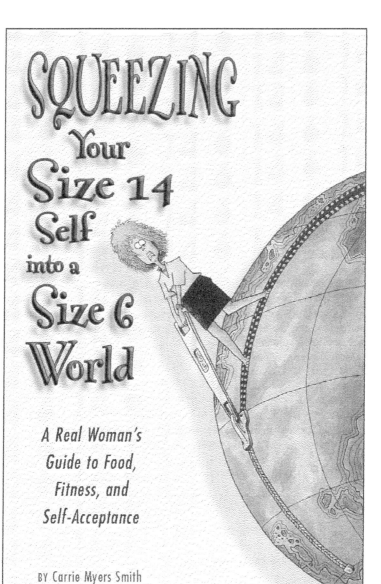

SQUEEZING
Your
Size 14
Self
into a
Size 6
World

*A Real Woman's
Guide to Food,
Fitness, and
Self-Acceptance*

BY Carrie Myers Smith

CHAMPION PRESS, LTD.
FREDONIA, WISCONSIN

Cover Illustration by Johnny Caldwell
Cover Design by Fineman Communications
Author Photograph by Jim Westphalen

ISBN: 1891400-304
LCCN: 2003110335

Manufactured in the United States of America 10 9 8 7 6

Dedication

To my five guys: my husband, Shawn, who is my biggest cheerleader and supporter, and my sons, Ericson, Marshall, Jackson, and Zachary, who help keep me accountable.

11/4/06

Diane —

To your wellness!

& Camille Salt

Small steps... big changes!

Acknowledgements

First and foremost, I'd like to thank my Lord and Savior, Jesus Christ, for allowing me the privilege of helping women reach their God-given potential, live by their passions, and realize what a gift their bodies are.

Thank you Sara Pattow, MaryAnn Koopmann, Brook Stowers, and Ginny Stephan for testing and growing my skills as a coach. You're all good friends and wonderful women—well on your way!

Thanks Mom and Dad for always expecting my best from me and for supporting my endeavors since childhood. I love you both!

Special thanks to Brook Stowers for believing in my (sometimes) crazy, far-fetched ideas, for your patience, your understanding and support, and your incredible insight. You're a truly amazing person, and I love you like a sister. One down, baby!

Finally, this project never would have gotten finished without the love, support and patience of my incredible husband, Shawn, and four sons, Ericson, Marshall, Jackson, and Zachary. You all sacrificed in some way to help make my dream possible. You guys are great! I'll love you always!

CONTENTS

Part Four:
Food, Fitness & You

Other Stuff

FOREWORD

In today's society it's almost impossible to feel good about your body, given the impossible standards we're expected to live up to. Airbrushed-to-perfection images in fashion magazines, actresses with body doubles—everywhere you look the message is clear: to be acceptable you have to be the perfect size 6. It's no wonder that 25-35 percent of college-aged women are engaging in binging and purging as weight management techniques. According to one American study, approximately 80-90 percent of women dislike their bodies. And a recent Canadian Gallup poll reported close to 70 percent of women are preoccupied with their weight—and almost 40 percent are perpetually dieting due to dissatisfaction with their appearance!

I've been where so many women still are today—trying desperately to fit the perfect mold. As a former model and actress, I found trying to meet the standards of the industry unhealthy—not to mention draining me of self-esteem. I never felt good enough. After having had enough, I left, and so began a journey of achieving true wellness. It hasn't always been easy, and it may not be for you, either. But with such an indispensable tool, such as this book, at your disposal, it's sure to ease your way and get you going down the path that's right for you.

With so many fitness and diet books out there, it's hard to know who believe—the information is so conflicting. One says to eat a low fat, high carbohydrate diet while another says a high protein, high fat, low carb diet is the way to lose weight.

It's confusing to say the least! What's more, none of these books actually looks at *why* you are eating; they only deal with *what*. And let's face it—ultimately it's not what you're eating, it's what's eating you! This is where *Squeezing Your Size 14 Self into a Size 6 World* stands head and shoulders above the crowd.

Getting to know yourself—what's eating you—is the basis to Carrie Myers Smith's concept. She takes you through simple step-by-step techniques, coaching you to a deeper understanding of what makes you feel and act the way you do. This book helps you see things from a different perspective by clearing away the "baggage" so you can move forward and grow from your experience.

Squeezing Your Size 14 Self into a Size 6 World de-mystifies food and fitness with easy-to-understand, up-to-date information on what you need to do to get fit and healthy through a balanced approach to nutrition, exercise, stress management, and self-nurturing. Carrie takes it one step further by looking at personality types and possible solutions for the typical problems that can be encountered on the road to true wellness. She then helps facilitate these changes by teaching you how to coach yourself with special "Coaching Moments" throughout the book. By learning these important coaching techniques, you will move easily through difficult situations. What's more, this book is full of helpful tips and inspirational quotes to help you stay motivated and moving toward your goals. *Squeezing Your Size 14 Self into a Size 6 World* helps you prepare for all the typical obstacles that can prevent you from reaching your goals and instills the importance of planning ahead.

Ultimately, this book teaches you how to accept yourself, regardless of your size. While it offers you easy-to-follow directions that will help you reach your aesthetic goals, you will also learn to love yourself on a whole new level—body, mind, and spirit. This is not just another diet book!

- Keli Roberts

ABOUT KELI ROBERTS:
Keli Roberts is the 2003 IDEA International Instructor of the Year and ACE Media Spokesperson. Known world wide for her award winning videos, books and training seminars, she specializes in strength and stability training, group exercise, personal training, and motivation. Keli holds certifications from the Australian Council for Health and Recreation, AFAA, ACE for group fitness and personal training and is also a BOSU Master Presenter, a Resist-A-Ball Master Trainer, a member of the Nautilus team and the Group Fitness Manager at Equinox in Pasadena.

INTRODUCTION

P erhaps you picked up this book with hesitation, because you're not a size 14, so you're not sure this book is for you. The average American woman is 5'4," 140 pounds, and a size 14—hence the title. And while this title is intended to refer to the average woman's size, it's really as much about a state of mind. You may be a size 4, but still struggle, trying to squeeze yourself into molds that don't fit you—and that ultimately, were never intended for you. And there are lots of them—molds that we, as women, attempt to squeeze into, from diets and fitness to other people's expectations and body image. And then, of course, there are the inevitable consequences to our act of squashing and squishing ourselves into some foreign form, including self-esteem issues and stress—lots of stress! You see, trying to squeeze into someone else's molds constricts you—it confines you to their rules—denying you the freedom of enjoying life and being the woman God intended for you to be.

Diets are a perfect example of this. Someone comes up with the "perfect" weight loss plan that magically fits everyone. And while you've tried every other "perfect" plan and failed, you think it can't hurt to try this one. After all, what have you got to lose—except hopefully, a few pounds? And so you go on the plan, and you feel good for the first couple of weeks. But then it begins to become monotonous. There are certain foods that aren't allowed on your menu, and entertaining—even feeding your own family—becomes increasingly difficult, as you have to prepare two different meals—one for you and one for them. There is no joy in eating. After a month or so, you've had it, and begin "cheating." You sneak forbidden foods—just a little at first, but the amount and frequency gradually increase, and before you know it, you've totally blown it and find yourself in a binge fest with your fridge. But what have you got to lose? Try another layer of your self-esteem.

This book attempts to address some of these issues, asking powerful questions throughout, so that you can come up with powerful answers that work for you and your life. *What do you mean so I can come up with the answers? I want you to give me the answers!* Let me explain. As a veteran in the fitness industry, one thing that has always bothered me has been our lack of success with the people who needed help the most. We seemed to mostly be making the fit fitter, but missing the mark with the unfit and sedentary. Fortunately, coaching has entered the scene. With its foundation in behavioral science, lifestyle, business, and now wellness coaches are helping people move from just surviving their lives to soaring through them.

Part of the basis of coaching is in asking questions to help the client set realistic goals and expectations. It is the coach's job to guide her client, not tell her what to do. While a coach may offer advice and options, it is ultimately the client who makes the decisions, sets her goals, and lays out her plan. It is, after all, the client who has to put the plan in motion, so doesn't it make sense that she should also design how to get there?

And that's the notion this book takes on. As a coach, I believe you probably need some guidance in certain areas of your life. As we all know, life sometimes has a way of just taking over. We feel as though we're just along for the ride, just out of grasp of the steering wheel. Or, perhaps you just need "permission" to break free of the molds you've been trying to squeeze into—just a gentle nudge to get you going—

like a mother horse nudges her colt up onto shaky, wobbly legs or a mother bird, her young fledgling out of the nest. I will offer you advice and options, but the plan is all yours. Try as you might, you won't find a prepackaged, nice, neat plan hidden between these covers. There is no "perfect" plan or agenda for you to photocopy, hang on your refrigerator door, and follow to the letter. There are no tricks intended to secretly trip you up.

There is, however, my hope, that you will find the beginning of a journey to true wellness—one that is tailor-made just for you.

There is one word of caution, however. Some of you may not be ready to begin this journey quite yet. Sometimes, we need to take a step or two backwards in order to move forward. As you read this book, determine if you are able to dump your old baggage and move forward from where you are right now. If you decide that you can't, then I encourage you to seek help from a qualified professional who can help you sort out past hurts and experiences, and how they are affecting your life today. This can be done in conjunction with your wellness plan, or you may need to work solely on just that. Either way, you will be taking the first step necessary in breaking free of the molds that have been confining you.

My Story

Before we jump into the book, I'd like to take a moment to tell you a little bit about myself. It's really important to me that you understand that I can relate to you. Often, we'll read a book and think, "What does this person really know? Sure, they've got the letters after their name, but does the label really equate to real life?" I admit—I often think this about parenting "experts," having four sons of my own! Sometimes, no amount of education can beat out real life experience!

I'm writing this book, because I am an "average" woman—not necessarily according to height and weight stats, but it's that mind-set thing. Growing up, I often felt the need to squeeze into other people's molds. I didn't feel the freedom to truly be myself—because if I did, would I be accepted? I believe that as humans, we have a tendency to slap on preconceived labels and stick people into certain stereotypical molds when it comes to certain attributes—whether it's what tax bracket they fall into, their IQ, their attractiveness quotient, their choice of career, their accent, or what part of town they come from. For me, I always felt I had to put a good face forward, never letting my true emotions peek through, or I was considered a "princess" and "spoiled brat." And a couple of "friends" told me so! So I squeezed and squeezed, trying to be whomever it was that people would (hopefully) like. And ouch! I still have the scars to prove it!

When we moved from our small town in Western NY to an even smaller town in Northern NH during my freshman year in high school, this need to be accepted increased exponentially. Being a pastor's kid, I was automatically labeled a "goody two shoes"—and boy, did I set out to smash that mold! While I won't go into too much detail—okay, *any* detail—over time, all this did was strip away, layer-by-layer, my self-esteem—what there was of it in the first place. In the end, I wasn't even sure who I was supposed to be or look like or how I was supposed to act. Eventually, in an attempt to gain some control in my life, I became anorexic. My attempt to gain control, however, ultimately became out of control.

My recovery from this eating disorder did not happen over night. It has been a long, slow, and at times, painful process— and a journey in rediscovering (or perhaps discovering for the first time!) who I am. I believe one reason I chose to enter the fitness field was because I could in many ways, use it to mask my disorder. As you'll soon read, those of us in the fitness industry don't come with a guarantee for high self-esteem or body image, nor are we immune from disordered eating and exercise patterns. At one point, I had to leave the industry that had become my safety net and comfort, in order to fully heal from the disorder.

Ultimately, however, the source of my true healing came from reconnecting to my God. I had made my "God connection" as a child, accepting Christ as my personal Savior at the age of twelve. However, I never nurtured that relationship and instead, became dependent on others' approval and acceptance for my self-esteem and self-worth. I also drew my self-esteem from my beauty and brains. But as I eventually found out, true self-esteem does not come from external, fleeting things—things that can be taken away from us at any time. Sure, these "things" can help us feel good about who we are, but ultimately, they cannot be our source of self-worth. Nor can we draw self-worth from ourselves, with techniques like positive self-talk. Yes, practical, hands-on tools will help, but they won't get to the core of the problem. By nurturing my relationship with God, through Christ, being secure in His unending, unconditional, unfailing love, and by doing practical applications like choosing to not buy into the media's perception of beauty, I have been able to accept myself for who I am—body and all. Does that mean I'm perfect? No way! Not even close! But I can love myself now, while at the same time, work on being my best no matter what my current situation. And you can, too. No matter where you are in your life, you can begin today to make the choice to start loving you—all of you—and to move forward in this journey called life. You can choose to stop squeezing yourself into molds that don't belong to you and start being the woman God created you to be. Hey! Life's a journey! Let's get going...

How to Use This Book

Throughout this book, you'll find little breaks in the text titled, "A Coaching Moment." These coaching moments are intended to help you more deeply reflect on the topic at hand. I highly recommend that you have a journal or notebook handy to copy down the questions and take the time to record thoughtful, meaningful responses. Or, if you'd like, there is a companion workbook to this book. In it are all the coaching moments, with room to record your thoughts. We've also included the other assignments and activities found throughout the book, and have cross-referenced everything. You can download the workbook by going to www.championpress.com. Or, buy the spiral-bound version, available wherever this book is found or at www.championpress.com.

PART ONE

Dumping Your Baggage

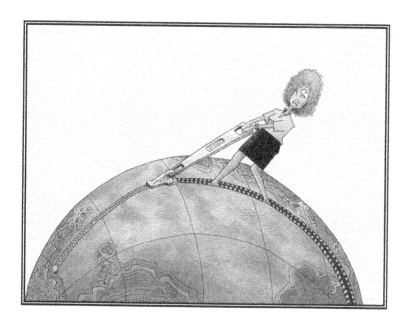

CHAPTER ONE

Your Ticket to Wellness

This journey is going to be different from any other you've ever taken before. Sure, it will be painful at times, but it's also going to be fun, joyful, freeing, and enlightening. If you're looking for the easy way out, still searching for that elusive magic pill or immediate gratification, then you might want to wait for the next bus. But, if you're looking to finally take a hammer to the body mold and become your own personal best, if a perfectionist mind-set is holding you captive, if the Superwoman "I-can-have-it-all-right-now-and-do-it-all-myself" syndrome is keeping you from having a joyful life, if you're sick and tired of being sick and tired due to your family's hectic schedules, then join us on our journey to a freer life. Are you ready? Then roll up your sleeves, grab your bags and let's get going!

That's the Ticket!

Just so I don't totally lose you in this next section, let me explain. We're taking a trip, a journey. Right? Well, on this journey, we're taking a motor home. Here, let me take a moment to set the scene. We're at your home—in your driveway, to be exact. Why, you ask, are we taking a motor home? Why not a plane or a train? They're much faster. Bingo. You answered your own question—they're faster. A motor home may not be the fastest mode of transportation, but that's exactly why we're taking it. Here, have a seat. We've got a few minutes before we leave (they're checking the oil and tire pressure). Get comfy and let me explain. A motor home is the vehicle of choice for several reasons. For starters, you can take a direct route to where you have to go. That's not possible with a plane, train, or bus. Sure, you can get a direct flight or route, but it's not exactly direct; you still have to take a cab from there to your destination. With a motor home, you can take stops when you need to—not on someone else's schedule. This allows you time to reflect and brainstorm, or just take a pit stop when you need to. And let's face it, it would take way too long to get your pilot's, engineer's, or bus driver's license (since you are the driver), and that would give you one more thing to procrastinate over.

But why can't I just take my car, you ask. *I already have my license for that.* Exactly. And look where it's gotten you! Besides, a motor home holds way more passengers, giving you plenty of supporters. And hey, the on-board bathroom is definitely a plus!

So now you know why we're taking a motor home, and just in time, too.

It's ready. Okay. Hop into the driver's seat. You want me to drive? Oh no! This is your journey. I'm just your guide. Now, grab your keys and let's go! What keys, you say? Here. You better sit back down. Listen. You've got the keys. You've had them all along. But you've allowed fear and self-doubt and feelings of unworthiness to take over. Other people's words and opinions have weighed you down. You've allowed the media's beauty ideals to determine how you feel about yourself. You know you'll never look as perfect as their images and it just eats you up. You feel smaller, more worthless, and even stupid at times. You try their diets and their workout plans, and you read or see the testimonies of women who do the programs and succeed, and you wonder why it doesn't work for you. What is wrong with you? It must be something you're doing. Right? Wrong! You have to stop depending on other people's opinions of you. You have to stop allowing society's ideals to be the barometer for how you feel about yourself. It does not matter what size your waist is. It does not matter what your dress size is. Your shoe size does not matter. Your bra size does not matter. Neither does the size of your nose, your paycheck, your house, or your bank account. Period. They do not matter. What *does* matter is the size of your heart and your ability to get past the self-focus, the obsessions and self-absorption, to see the bigger picture.

There is a wonderful children's book that illustrates "special-ness" perfectly. The book is *You Are Special* by Max Lucado. It is a parable-type story that tells about wooden people named Wemmicks (who symbolize us), carved by Eli, their woodworker, and is a reflection of our own lives. Now, the Wemmicks have a strange ritual; they stick stickers on each other: golden star stickers for those Wemmicks who "deserve it"—they're either beautiful or tall or talented—and gray circle stickers on those "bad" Wemmicks—those who don't meet their society's

> "Remember," Eli said as the Wemmick walked out the door, "you are special because I made you. And I don't make mistakes."
>
> ...from *You are Special*
> by Max Lucado

standards. The story centers around Punchinello, a poor Wemmick who never seems to say or do the right thing. Oh, and he wasn't blessed with good looks, and to top it all off, his wood is becoming all scratched and gouged. He meets a Wemmick one day named Lucia, who has no stickers on her. She's "different." This really catches Punchinello's attention, since he's never seen a Wemmick without stickers before! So he asks her about it. Seems she's been spending some time with Eli. And because of this, the other Wemmicks' stickers don't stick to Lucia anymore. Try as they might, the stickers slide right off. She encourages Punchinello to go visit Eli, too—says he's even expecting him. It takes a day or so, but Punchinello does make his way up the hill to Eli's cottage-workshop. Reluctantly, he enters and is immediately greeted with a warm welcome.

Punchinello is shocked that Eli knows his name. Eli responds that of course he knows his name—he made him! Punchinello asks Eli about Lucia and inquires about why stickers don't stick to her. Is she using some special moisturizing oil or something? Eli responds that it's because Lucia cares more about what Eli thinks than what the other Wemmicks think about her. And she visits Eli every day.

Punchinello still didn't understand, but Eli told him he would, and encouraged him to stop by and visit every day. As

> While it's easy to get caught up in our day-to-day craziness and chaos, he-said-she-said, what have I done wrong now, self-defeating head games, remember that you *choose* to live that way.

Punchinello was leaving, he was thinking about what Eli said, trying to grasp the meaning. And while he didn't fully understand it yet, he believed Eli when he said that Punchinello was special to him. And as he thought that thought, one of his stickers fell off.

You are special... no matter what. And you are worth just as much as someone 100 pounds lighter or 100 pounds heavier. While it's easy to get caught up in our day-to-day crazy and chaotic, he-said-she-said, what have I done wrong now, self-defeating head games, remember that you *choose* to live that way. There is another way and through this book, I hope to share it with you. But before we can move forward, we need to make sure that you aren't bringing extra baggage. On this trip we have a zero bag limit. I know you get to check two on the plane and all... but we have a lot of passengers to fit and no extra room! Trust me, we don't need extra baggage on this journey. So let's take a look at what baggage you have been toting around all these years.

CHAPTER TWO

In Search of Barbie®...
(or *does she exist?*)

One big ol' bag of garbage that we carry around is our body—and specifically, our perception of it. Tell me—how many Barbies® did you have as a little girl? I think I had two, plus Ken, of course (although, don't ask me how I thought it was okay for him to have two women!). I also had many accessories—clothes (many of which my great grandmother sewed or knit), shoes, purses, jewelry, and the pool. I'm not even sure it was an official Barbie® pool, since it was a blow-up version, but it worked for me. I loved to go to my friend's house down the street and play Barbies®. Oh...she had everything Barbie®, including the Town House, sports car, and the official Malibu pool—patio and all. But as I think about it all now, I wonder why there is such a fascination with Barbie®. I think it's probably because she's just so...perfect. And being little girls, playing with her, we could be her, and live vicariously through her. When we're little girls, we can pretend we have the perfect body, the perfect mate, the perfect house, the perfect life. And we can dream about how, when we're grown, our own lives will be just that, too—perfect. And then we hit puberty.

"It is easy to say that Barbie® has had nothing to do with women deciding to have breast implants or starve themselves to death. It is also just as easy to put all the blame on her. Unfortunately, there has been so much emphasis on blame that the real issues about this larger-than-life icon have become an argument for the media.

I do not believe that my grandmother had any idea how Barbie® would take the world by storm; if she were still in the driver's seat, I believe there would be 'heavy' Barbie® and Stacie® dolls on the market today. The question is: Would the majority of the population buy them? Therein lies the problem. So Barbie® lovers can rest easy: Barbie® is not to blame, we are. As a society, we buy into this perfect image that has been placed as a mental burden on the shoulders of women everywhere."—from *The Body Burden: Living in the Shadow of Barbie* by Stacey Handler, granddaughter to the original creator of Barbie® and namesake to the Stacie® doll

Remember that geeky, gangly stage we hit around age eleven? We started tripping over our own two feet and couldn't get out of our own way? We think, "This can't last long, this feeling like I'm being taken over by aliens." But then it gets worse. We start "blossoming," and it isn't long before we're standing at the bra counter, while our mother discusses lace, underwires, or practicality. But we still have hope. I mean, Barbie® has boobs and look at her. The problem is, as we're developing, we're gaining more than just breasts. We're getting padding in places Barbie® doesn't have it. Then we begin looking beyond just Barbie®. Magazine covers are garnished with teenage girls and women who, while they may have breasts, that's about all they have. And so the downward spiral begins. While most of us think we gave up Barbie® long ago, chances are, we're still holding on to her. She may go by a different name—Nikki, Kate, Tyra—but it's still the same image: perfect breasts, slim hips, tiny waist, and endless legs. From television, to movies, to magazines, we're constantly bombarded by images of beautiful women—some exotic, some wholesome, some gorgeous, always "perfect," always the same end result. We put ourselves down. We say we're not good enough. We'll never measure up. Some of us wallow in our sorrow by burying our faces in a carton of ice cream (make mine New York Super Fudge Chunk, please!). After all, if we'll never be those images, then why try at all?

Others die trying. We workout every second we can, replacing other things in our lives with this obsessive need to workout. We replace shopping with a friend, with going for a run. Dinners out with family are replaced by going to the gym. A movie date with our husband is replaced by endless sit-ups and leg raises. Time spent relaxing is replaced by total anxiety over not working out that specific moment. And so the cyclic torturing continues—over what? Over images that in all likelihood aren't even real.

A Coaching Moment

Stop and think a moment about your "Barbie" perceptions. If you could design the "perfect" body, what would it be? Go ahead—list it all out. Now compare your body to your "perfect" body. Do both bodies have arms for hugging your loved-ones and legs to carry you on your journey? Do both bodies have an intelligent, thinking brain and a strong, beating heart? Do the aesthetic differences really matter when you consider the true, functional purposes of our bodies? Why?

"As a hefty size 14, I often hear people tell me, 'You are not a plus-size.' Everaything's relative. If you were to put me next to a standard-size model, I would be about six sizes bigger than she is. Most of the models you see in advertising and editorial photographs are size 2 to 8, wearing size 8 clothing, which is the sample-size standard. (You should see how the clothes are pinned in the back!)

Welcome to 'fashion reality.' Just as I, as a size 14 represent the 'plus-size' woman, models who are tall, slim, and small-boned represent the 'average' American woman. The real average American woman is actually 5'4," about 140 pounds, and a size 14.

In the fashion business, 'reality' is often not depicted realistically. That's true, by the way, not only with regard to size. In many fashion photographs, stray hairs are routinely airbrushed out, as are shadows, wrinkles, blemishes, and even freckles. And that's after the hair and makeup people have finished with the models! In both fashion and beauty—as in Hollywood—perfection is the reality."

—*Natalie Laughlin,*
www.natalielaughlin.com

In response to an interviewer's question regarding weight gain and loss of celebrities:
"I'm not so sure that it's *people* who are obsessed with the weight of celebrities or the *media* that's obsessed. You're damned if you're too thin and you're damned if you're too heavy." —Jennifer Aniston, *Redbook*, August, 2001

Joan Lunden recently did an episode of "Behind Closed Doors" where she discusses the fashion and magazine industries and what goes on, well, behind closed doors. It's a real eye-opener, and in case you missed it, I'll review some of the info here.

So how do they make a cover photo? Throw the clothes on the model, take the picture, and copy it a million times on the cover of the magazine? If only it were true, then at least we would have something real to be jealous over! The magazines want you to believe this perfect body does exist (part of the head games, which we'll cover in our next chapter). Or as a fashion director for *Cosmo* says in the "Behind Closed Doors" segment, "That's what a fashion picture is all about. It has to look *perfect* (emphasis added) on the page so that every girl who sees that outfit will want to go out and buy it."

I have a few issues with this. First of all, many of the outfits you see on the cover of magazines are one-of-a-kind, straight-off-the-runway. So if there's only one, how can anyone else get it? Secondly, most of the time half the dress is missing! Where would you wear something that barely covered your chest, let alone your mid-section? Thirdly, this fashion director admitted that they are trying to create a perfect look. How they do it is even more interesting...

According to another one of the professionals on the tape, it comes down to making the person fit the dress. "You can really make anything *perfect* (emphasis added), whether it's a subtle change or a master, big change," she says.

The tools of the trade? Try a variety of tape, including duct and surgical, pads, girdles, bras, shapers, and cinchers. Since the outfits the models wear come in only one standard size, the stylists literally make the models fit the clothing as much as they make the clothing fit the model. They want the outfit to hang perfectly on the body— not too tight, not too loose. So they clothespin the back of it, or duct tape it, pin it, or tie it, or they use these big, heavy clamps, which pull the fabric down and help it to hang "just right." Of course, we can't see any of this, because we see only the front of the model. How many cover photos are taken of the model looking back at you? Not many. If they were, they would be pinned up the front!

> In an August 2001 *Redbook* interview, Jennifer Aniston was asked why she's involved with a teen girl's web site, Voxxy.com. Her response: "I think it is important to demystify the celebrity thing for young girls. All these beauty magazines, including this one, need to be more responsible with what you feed young girls. They don't know that it takes hours to do hair and makeup for a photo shoot, and that then some computer is used to take off the pimple on your face and erase stray hairs and extra curves. It sets an impossible standard for these young girls to live up to. I realize that the magazines need to sell and there is pressure for perfecting an image on the covers, but I want young girls to know it's not real— it's magic!"

Okay, now let's say the model doesn't have too much up front. Her breasts can be lifted using surgical tape, or padded by using silicon padding—whichever works for the look they're trying to achieve. Not much in the rear end? No problem. Or at least nothing that either an elasticized butt booster or LYCRA® padding won't help. Need to cinch in that waist (remind you of another era? Can you say corset?)? A waist whittler is just what the doctor ordered. The key, say experts, is to create a "proportioned look."

Once the model is "perfected" and the photo shoot done, the picture is ready to go, right? Yeah, right—ready to go right on to Nashville, Tennessee, but not for it's country music debut. A company that specializes in photo retouching receives the chosen cover photo—which, by the way, has already been dissected-apart and mapped-out by the magazine editors, so that the computer technicians know which parts need to be perfected—and feeds the photo into a digital scanner which then in turn feeds the image into a retouching computer. Yep. They've actually got a special computer whose only job is to touch-up photos. "There's almost nothing that we can't fix, I mean, the possibilities are endless," says the company representative. "We're creating a reality. It's the virtual reality of magazine publishing."

Did you catch that? A virtual reality. What we see in these magazines isn't even real!

As an example, in the video, they show how a cover photo of Cindy Crawford was retouched. Yeah. Even Cindy Crawford is perfected! In this one photo they used airbrushing to soften tones and shadows, trimmed off the back of her arms, smoothed out the wrinkles in her dress, erased the lines off her hands, and carved off several inches from her thighs—"excess baggage," according to the host, due to a bad camera angle. A "radical redo" of a photo can take a whole day and up to $10,000! But it doesn't end there. They can even take different body parts—the parts they consider to fit the perfect mold— and put them together. So you may see Model A's head, but her body may actually belong to Model B.

Fashion magazines aren't the only ones who attempt to project the perfect image. Even health and fitness magazines aren't immune.

"Yes, we definitely Photoshop," comments one editor from a health and fitness magazine.

"Sometimes it's minor things, like taking out nipples here and there, but we've made people taller, boobs smaller, created different outfits for models...sometimes smiles are too wide and clown-like, and they make them smaller. Sometimes hair is too crazy, and they tone it down. I have seen them take a head from one picture and put it on a different body! I am really trying to keep the intense Photoshop work down, but they always adjust skin tones, and have gotten rid of sweat stains in unsightly places as well. It's a fine line, I have to agree. And unfortunately misleading for women at times."

"It is a conundrum we all face in participating in the problem," adds another former editor, "and the editors on staff do, too. But it's the head honcho—editor-in-chief—and the art director—who usually influences her—who most definitely direct the tone and visual messages of the magazine. Even if lowlier editors disagree they can't do anything about it—they don't have the ultimate say in images or words."

I want you to get the true, full effect of what is being said here, so I'm going to let you "listen in" to a conversation I had with this former editor. Check this out:

"[At one point, I] had direct orders not to choose fit models—prior to [this editor-in-chief arriving], I would audition all the models we cast for exercise shoots to make sure they could actually do squats, lift five pound dumbbells, etc. All that ended because we were told to use 'fashiony' (i.e. skinny) models instead. This was meant to give the magazine a more trendy feel and attract more advertisers."

I remember one time for an upper body/arm workout I was totally alarmed because the 'opener' shot was an anorexic model 'flexing' a nonexistent bicep. She was a skeleton and I pointed this out and said there was no way we could use this picture to promote building upper body strength. It took [the editor-in-chief] a while to see my point, but eventually she had the art department 'Photoshop' in a little more flesh to create somewhat more of a curve.

The problem with catering to advertisers is that to some degree much of the fashion/beauty world (among the biggest advertisers) is filled with 'artsy' types and all that image connotes is true in my experience: very few models, photographers, hair people, stylists, makeup people, and art/graphic designers, exercise or eat well. They smoke a lot, and if they do any activity they might do yoga because it's trendy and fashionable, but very few are really into fitness. I find this on photo shoots all the time.

> "Part of it *is* giving the readers what they say they don't want, but still buy."

And so their image of what's attractive is very, very different. Anyway, you can't wear much high-end fashion unless you're really thin and have no muscles. Ever try slipping a pair of Jimmy Choo boots over runner's calves? Or any cool pants these days over muscular thighs? And that whole world feeds off of itself. And celebrities and designers and yadda yadda. So these same attitudes carry over with the editors that want to be a part of that world (and if you notice the direction that [many fitness magazines] have gone to—very fashiony—you can see the yearning to make the magazine be aligned with that world).

On the other hand, of course, more readers read this kind of stuff than some of the smaller, more fitness-oriented magazines. Part of it is giving the readers what they say they don't want, but still buy."

A Coaching Moment

How do you really feel about the models on the covers of magazines? How does it make you feel about your own body seeing stick-thin models who supposedly represent the "average" woman? Are you supporting publications and products that make you feel bad about yourself? What benefits are you gaining?

Which Came First: The Eating Disorder or The Aerobics Instructor?

Models and actresses aren't the only ones who feel intense pressure to slim down. As fitness has become more commercialized, fitness professionals, including group fitness instructors (the modern term for the good ol' aerobics instructor) and personal trainers, have been prodded to follow suit. Studies show a rise in eating disorders amongst group fitness instructors. This doesn't surprise me. When I taught aerobics in college, there was this unspoken competition among the instructors with our bodies. You know how women are when we "check each other out." Do we hoot and holler or whistle and cackle? No! We're discrete. We can walk by another woman with barely a glance and still get her approximate weight, height, body fat percentage, bust-waist-hip measurements—heck, we can tell what she ate for breakfast, whether she colors her hair, and whether or not "those" are real. Right? Imagine the tension when a whole group of instructors gathered for a staff meeting. I'm sure I wasn't the only one who ran all the way home after the meeting and worked out for another two hours. After all, we are the examples, the role models, of health and fitness. Instructors are standing up in front of rooms of participants who expect them to look the part. The pressure can be intense—whether it's pressure put upon themselves, or coming from outside sources doesn't matter. The end result is the same. Many healthy role models are delving into unhealthy behaviors and attitudes.

In a study done at Coastal Carolina University in Conway, South Carolina, 368 female group fitness instructors completed a survey which covered the following areas: eating disorders, maladaptive eating attitudes, obligatory exercise (a compulsion to exercise beyond normal frequency and/or duration,

---

CCU Study Results
Number of Respondents: 368

Previous Eating Disorder: 21%
Maladaptive Eating Attitudes: 6%
Obligatory Exercise: 4.1%
Body Dissatisfaction: 42.9% wanted to be thinner
Weight Management Practices: 37.3% said they were currently trying to lose weight

---

regardless of social or physical consequences), body dissatisfaction, and weight management practices.

According to this study, based on their BMI (body mass index, a measurement of weight to height) five percent of the respondents fell in the underweight category and 85.1 percent were of average weight. Compare these numbers to the number who were dissatisfied with their bodies and with the number trying to lose weight. What I find especially interesting is that compared to the average population, the percentage of instructors with past (and very possibly present) eating disorders is much higher (compare 21 percent with 5-10 percent!). According to the survey results, most of the instructors with a previous eating disorder (80.3 percent) said they had the condition prior to teaching classes. This would seem to answer the question, "Which came first: the eating disorder or the aerobics instructor?" It appears women with a history of an eating disorder are drawn to the business of fitness—such as I was.

Other studies show similar results. In research done at the University of Montgomery, Alabama, 40 percent of the female instructors surveyed reported a history of disordered eating. In a follow-up study done four years later, instructors under 30 years of age showed more body-image dissatisfaction than

Body mass index (BMI) is basically just a height/weight chart. While it can give you a ballpark estimate of health risk, it's not as accurate as body composition. I also want to steer you away from immersing yourself in so many numbers, and to especially pull you away from the scale. We'll discuss more of this in the second half of the book, but for now, let's begin to grasp a fresh perspective!

instructors over 30 years of age—even though they had below-average body fat percentages. And researchers at Indiana University found that 44 percent of the 250 female instructors in their study could be classified as obligatory exercisers.

But eating disorders are just a part of the unhealthy world of our supposedly healthy role models. A friend of mine tells of fitness-conference participants and speakers who take smoke breaks. My guess is that the smoking keeps the pounds off—a common reason that actresses smoke. What is that doing, though, besides trading one bad habit for another? Then there are the nutritional supplements, many of which today contain appetite suppressors and "fat burners." These are nothing more than modern day diet pills. Oh, but it gets better. When all this doesn't squeeze us into the mold, there is always—ta da—ab etching. Sort of like an Etch A Sketch®, but for your abs! Actually, it's a form of liposuction, where the surgeon creates the much sought-after six-pack look. You know, the washboard abs? But it's not just men who want this look, it's women, too. According to a Manhattan surgeon's press release, "Ab-etching is now the trade secret of fitness trainers who, years ago would not be caught dead in a plastic surgeon's office. With pressure for personal trainers to 'look the part' and be their 'buff best,' they, too, often resort to cosmetic surgery and in particular, this method of liposuction."

> My biggest concern is that those resorting to surgery are still preaching the healthy stuff, and keeping their surgery a secret. In this case, they then become false advertisements, placing even greater pressure on consumers to attain the unattainable.

So not only are some fitness professionals engaging in unhealthy, sometimes, potentially dangerous behaviors, but they're resorting to plastic surgery to try to attain the perfect body. What does that say about fitness today? And what kind of role models are today's fitness professionals? Sure, many, if not most, are good role models, but unfortunately, more and more are turning to aberrant behaviors to try to meet their own unattainable goal. Perhaps most disturbing of all is, where is the integrity in all of this? As fitness professionals, we promote healthy eating, exercise, and stress reduction. Should we also be promoting—or in some cases advertising—plastic surgery? My biggest concern is that those resorting to surgery are still preaching the healthy stuff, and keeping their surgery a secret. In this case, they then become false advertisements, placing even greater pressure on consumers to attain the unattainable.

"The beauty culture confuses so many health issues. Thinness is confused with fitness. Well-applied cosmetic artifice is passed off as health. Anorexic models pose in sports equipment they are too weak to use. Women diet their breasts away then 'correct' the 'condition' with implant surgery. 'Sexy' is defined in body fat percentages too low for fertility or libido. We read health and fitness tips from models who admit they never work out.

A culture obsessed with artificial thinness, giddy with the power to dictate the 'appropriate' female form, has misappropriated women's desire to be simply healthy. The otherwise worthy goal of fitness is turned into yet another elusive beauty goal. In the cult of fitness chic, it is not enough to be fit and strong; a woman must also look slinky in a leotard.

In fact, in the world of Beautiful Fitness, if all she does is look slinky in the leotard she is assumed to be fit and healthy!"

"It is great that sports and fitness are more accessible and available to women today, but unfortunately the beauty culture has introduced frustrating, paradoxical ideals; a woman must be thin, taut, and muscular, but not 'too' muscular. She must strive for low body fat (often far too low for a healthy woman) but still have large breasts. A woman who is extremely fit but still has female fat distribution is diagnosed with 'unhealthy' extra weight. Often, top female athletes only receive mass media coverage if they 'look pretty' as well.

The twisted message of the 'fitness will make you beautiful' craze is that being fit, healthy, and strong will help a woman become beautiful, but she can prove her fitness only by becoming beautiful. The result is exercise fashions, exercise makeup and locker-room beauty anxiety. The garbled message is not 'fitness is beautiful,' which would make every woman potentially beautiful, but instead 'beautiful fitness is beautiful,' leaving us baffled again.

Is it any wonder you may feel depressed and resentful about pursuing your health goals, or confused about whether fitness is worth the effort if you don't become 'regulation beautiful?' Fitness is not the problem. Beautiful Fitness is the problem. Fitness feels powerful, wonderful. Beautiful Fitness feels frustrating and contributes to eating disorders and compulsive over-exercising.

Fitness is fitness. Fitness is beautiful. Beautiful Fitness is a manipulative fantasy of the beauty culture. You can tell the difference, and you can make the choice." —*The Mass Market Woman: defining yourself as a person in a world that defines you by your appearance* by Linda McBryde, M.D.

It wasn't long after I finished college that I felt I had to get out of the fitness industry. Here I was, I had just finished a degree in exercise science, and I had already had enough. I was trying to heal from anorexia, but being in the fitness environment was throwing me against the wall, instead of offering solace. I felt like I would never measure up as a true fitness professional. Trying to do so was just reviving bad habits. So I quit—temporarily. I quit teaching fitness classes and training. I cancelled my health club membership, cancelled my professional memberships, and my professional subscriptions. I also cancelled my fitness magazine subscriptions. Seeing all those "role models" of fitness was too much to take. I mean, do most of those models even workout? And if they did, where was the muscle to show for it? All I saw was half-starved women weakly smiling out from a magazine cover.

I did obviously ease back into the fitness field, but not until I had time to heal. The reason I bring all this up is to show that "role models" or "fitness idols" may be just virtual realities. You can't always tell just by looking, whether someone is starving herself or going home after class and binging until she

> Researchers are starting to take a look at what effect fitness magazines have on women and girls. Researchers at Brigham Young University surveyed 500 high school girls about their exercise and weight-loss methods. The girls who used diet pills, laxatives, vomiting, or restricted diets to lose weight were more likely than their non-dieting peers to read health and fitness magazines.

has to purge. You can't tell just by looking at her if she's taking fat burning pills—or worse, drugs—to keep her weight down. And you can't tell just by looking, if she's seeing a plastic surgeon to suck out fat that could be genetically impossible to get rid of otherwise. You see, many fitness professionals today preach one thing—healthy living, eating, exercise—but hold themselves to a different standard. Likewise, magazines often write about health, yet use unhealthy models as illustrations. And if these women can't attain the "ideal" naturally, they often turn to other methods.

We all need to stop using other women as our mold. Sure, we can admire other bodies, but let's stop there. We can feel admiration for others' bodies without hating our own bodies for their differences.

Begin today to change your thought process, separating reality from make-believe. Today is the day to start loving who you are!

A Coaching Moment

Who are your role models? What about each one of these people makes him or her a beautiful person? What do you believe makes you a beautiful person? What about yourself would you change if you could? Is this a realistic change? Is it worth the price?

Stepping Stones

- Barbie® is not a real woman.
- Most magazine images are fake.
- Stop basing your reality on fantasy.
- Comparing yourself to other women is futile.
- Celebrate our differences rather than envy them.

CHAPTER THREE

Check Your Baggage at the Door, Please

Okay. Everyone got your bags ready? First stop: the landfill. Please form a single line. No pushing or shoving. Follow me. What? You don't want to get rid of all that old baggage? Ah. All those past hurts are too precious, aren't they? All that unforgiveness and bitterness forms a nice little wall of protection, doesn't it? It also gives us a reason to eat and eat and not nurture ourselves since the added weight is just that much more protection, right? What? You'd rather go next door to the recycling center? Nope. That won't work. You see, when we take our old baggage and recycle it, it may look like something new, but it's still old garbage—just newly repackaged. If you're going to join this journey, you need to start fresh, start over, without all that old mucky-muck. It just goops everything up and gets in the way of the woman God intended you to be. You've got to be willing to take risks, make mistakes, get dirty—but also be willing to stand up, dust yourself off (or take a power shower, depending on how deep the mud was!), and continue on. While some may think this is simplifying it too much (and hey, that's one thing we're here for—simplification, right?), I feel that many changes can really

> When we take our old baggage and recycle it, it may look like something new, but it's still old garbage—just newly repackaged.

be boiled down to a four-step process: desire, choose, plan, and act. Before we go back to the motor home, let's walk together…

A Coaching Moment

What kind of old baggage are you holding onto? Will you allow old hurts and unforgiveness to hold you back from being the woman you were intended to be? What do you need to do to get rid of your old baggage?

Baby Steps

The first step in starting a lifestyle of wellness is to really want or desire it. While at first glance, this doesn't seem necessary for many things in our lives—I hate to grocery shop, for instance—there is still an underlying desire—some sort of end result that is desired regardless of whether or not we like the process of getting there. For instance, even though I can't stand the whole (what seems like) day-long process of grocery shopping—the list making, the coupon clipping, the getting everyone out the door and loaded into the mini-van, the drive, the shopping, then loading everything into the van only to unload the whole thing upon arrival home, and finally, putting it all away…only to have it used up, listening to everyone complain that there's nothing to eat, and having to start the process all over again the next week (and I didn't even mention the cost of it all!)—I still have a strong desire to eat healthy and feed my family decent meals. I can't say as I love to do dishes or laundry—my two other nemeses—but I do have a desire to eat from clean dishes and have clean clothes to wear. I also don't like the clutter dirty dishes make all over my counter, or when it appears the laundry bomb has gone off in my house. So while I don't necessarily enjoy the process of "getting there," I do have worthy, healthy desires. I can also change my attitude about the process, which we'll discuss later in the book.

This same type of idea applies to living a lifestyle of wellness. You've got certain wellness-related desires, whether they're something more general, like to live a long, healthy life or something more specific, like avoiding diabetes, heart disease, cancer, or osteoporosis. You can then develop a wellness plan, designing your goals based on your desires. Developing goals based on your desires increases your motivation—you've got a reason *why* you're doing what you're doing—and your incentive—you'll see a pay-off by being healthier and feeling better.

A Coaching Moment

What are your underlying reasons for wanting to live a healthy life?

But I hate the process of getting there! you say. As I said before, part of the solution to this is changing your attitude about the process, which we'll discuss later. Another piece of this puzzle is designing your plan around your preferences— not someone else's. It all goes back to the mold thing. For years, you've been trying to squeeze into someone else's mold—but that mold never was intended for you! If you've truly got the desire to live a lifestyle of wellness, then you will be able to develop a plan for getting there and a way to enjoy doing so (for the most part!). If you don't truly desire a healthier life—body, mind and spirit—you need to ask yourself if you're truly deep-down, spirit-filled, happy and satisfied with where you're at right now in your life. If your answer is yes, then keep on keeping on (and go give this book to someone who can really use it!)! But if it's no, then you need to ask what it is that's holding you back from the life you could be having.

A Coaching Moment
What changes do you desire in your life?

Chances are your answer is related in some way to fear, in which case, you may still have the desire to change buried somewhere down there, but fear has been overriding it. Be careful not to confuse fear with lack of desire. You can want something, but be fearful of the process. Fear is a normal human emotion, but one that can often derail our desires if we let it. We allow our fear to take over and it then becomes so ominous that we say, "Forget it. It's not worth the risk or the effort." It stops us in our tracks and we end up settling for where we are. But we need to remember that bravery is not a lack of fear. It is having the courage to plod ahead, despite being afraid. Do you think those firefighters and policemen who ran into the Twin Towers on 9/11 weren't afraid? The difference is, they didn't let the fear overtake them and their purpose. They knew they had a job to do and they did it—despite the risk.

> Be careful not to confuse fear with a lack of desire. You can want something, but be fearful of the process.

And you also have a job to do—to take care of yourself and live up to your potential, despite whatever risk may be involved, no matter what obstacles you're bound to run into (sometimes literally!).

A Coaching Moment

Is fear holding you back from making your desired changes? How will you release that fear so that you can move ahead in your journey?

Bridge Over Troubled Waters

Choosing to change is the bridge that connects wanting to change and actually taking action. It bridges our minds and hearts to our hands and feet. It takes us to the next step. But before we cross this bridge you should know what's in store for you. You see, once you come to the Bridge of Change, you need to make a decision: will you stay where you are? Or will you move forward? Will you stubbornly plant your feet and ignore your heart's desire to change and your purpose in life? Or will you cross this bridge? If you choose to stay where you are, then you may as well get on a bus and head back home. Oh, and there is no complaining or whining allowed. You have the tools to change at your disposal and I'll give you more throughout this book. Whining and

> Remember that bravery is not a lack of fear! It is having the courage to move forward, despite being afraid.

complaining is like taking a detour through six feet of mud. Take the high road—it's much easier. Of course, your motor home is always available. So if you change your mind, fill'er up and hop on!

If you choose to cross this bridge I must warn you that it will be painful and scary at times. There are trolls living under this bridge—ones who will try to stop you. Trolls who will do anything and everything in their power to knock you off the bridge or to scare you and make you run back to "safety." That's

> "At every moment we are choosing either to reveal ourselves or to protect ourselves, to value ourselves or to diminish ourselves, to tell the truth or to hide. To dive into life or to avoid it. Intimacy is making the choice to be connected to, rather than isolated from, our deepest truth at that moment."
> —Excerpted from, *When Food is Love: Exploring the Relationship Between Eating and Intimacy*, by Geneen Roth Plume, 1992

okay. If you do turn around and run or even fall off and get all wet, you simply start over again at desire. Re-evaluate how much you want this change. In some cases, it will go even beyond desire. It will be a need. You need to change to live. Use this time to come up with a plan. And while you do, take one step at a time over the bridge. For some women, the slow baby steps process doesn't work. They need to run across that bridge in leaps and bounds. But for others, the process is slower. They need time to test the waters to make sure this is the right thing to do. Your decision on which approach to take may also depend on how your decision will affect others, especially your family. Whichever approach you take, however, it's still one step at a time—whether it's done at a sprinter's pace or a snail's.

Between choosing and taking action is planning. While many people skip this step or feel it's unnecessary, I believe in planning wholeheartedly. If you don't plan how you're going to get over those inevitable obstacles, you will end up running straight into them, falling flat on your face. Depending on your personality, you may or may not get up and try again. And even if you do try again, without a plan, you will just be asking history to repeat itself. We'll discuss gracefully leaping your hurdles later in the book.

A Coaching Moment

Do you tend to skip the planning stage? What do you need to do to slow down long enough to plan ahead?

Taking action to change is the last step. Let's put this into practical language and something we can all relate to: chocolate. As I sit here writing this, I want some chocolate. Period. I want some. I crave it. But I don't have to go any further than that. As you can see, wanting something is pretty passive. You think it, but you don't have to act upon it. Now I'm going to choose to have chocolate. Choosing is a bit more active than simply wanting it. It involves me making more of a conscious choice to have the chocolate. I also have to choose and plan which kind to have: milk chocolate, dark, white, with nuts, without nuts, and if with nuts, what kind. As I sit here, however, I don't currently have all these options. I am at the mercy of whatever is available in my cupboard. (It's dark. No nuts.) I also have to plan out how to get it without my kids noticing, because they'll be all over me asking for some. Timing is key! They all have to be in just the right positions in the other room, not within eye-shot of seeing me open the cupboard (yeah—we've got one of those cupboards—the one where the goodies are stashed!), and they need to be making enough noise so they don't hear the wrapper. Of course, I never know when one of them may be headed on through to the other end of the house, so I also have to plan ahead as to how I will hide it from them if they do in fact choose that route. You see why planning is imperative? Now, after my plan is in place, I must act on my desire and choice to have chocolate. I'll get up, go to the cupboard and take the chocolate—and of course, eat it.

This type of thought process goes on in our minds all the time, but we're usually on autopilot. To establish new habits, it needs to be a bit more conscious. We need to plan, plan and plan!

There's also a process for more cognitive or spiritual aspects that is even more simplified than the procedure we go through when we're making a behavioral change. When we're presented with a concept, we can choose to accept it or choose to reject it. Choice is the main step in this process, because when we sift away everything else, all that's left is a choice— to believe or not believe.

I run into this with my clients quite often, especially in the area of self-worth. Through the years, we've conditioned ourselves to believe a certain way, usually that we're not worthy of or don't deserve certain things. "I don't deserve time to myself," says one mother. "I'm not worthy of anyone's love," an unmarried single woman convinces herself. "I'm worthless," says another very successful woman, who, while she's confident in what she can do, has no self-esteem in who she simply is.

A Coaching Moment

In what areas of your life do you lack confidence? Do you feel you have self-worth, right down to your core, simply because you are you? What is your basis for this belief?

In cases such as this, where it's not necessarily a behavior that needs to be changed, but an attitude, it boils down to a choice. You can choose to believe you are worth taking care of...or you can continue down the same stagnant path you've been on. This concept is what I've had to finally present to some of my clients, after trying all the "self-help" suggestions.

Let's face it. If you choose to believe you're dirt, no amount of self-care, self-pampering, or self-nurturing will dig that ugly core out of you. You'll be shiny on the outside, but you'll still be full of dirt on the inside. Until you accept that fact that you weren't put here on this earth by accident—that God didn't make some cosmic mistake by allowing you to take that first breath of air—you will never really have true self-esteem. You must make that connection—the "God connection"—to fully come to terms with your humanness and specialness. And if you believe what the Bible says, that connection will be made through Christ.

Maybe you've already made the connection, but still feel worthless inside. You say you believe it, but are you living it? We all say we want the joy and peace we see in some people. Have you ever thought about the difference between you and them? There's a difference between giving lip service—saying you believe something—and actually living it. Any activist will tell you that. There are those who say they support some cause—then there are those who do something about it. And within the doers, there are different facets of doing—all important, all necessary, none more important than the others—just different. It goes right back to that action step. If you say you've made that God-connection through Christ, but don't live it, what good is that? If you've really made that connection, you have no excuse not to believe you're worth taking care of. Stop trashing your temple! It's a choice! Believe that you should take care of yourself, choose to stop squeezing yourself into some mold (or totally rebelling altogether and going in the opposite direction), and take action to make it happen. Quite frankly (and I'm going to throw in a little tough love here), there are a lot of physically unfit Christians. Have you noticed? Maybe you're one of them. I don't know the reasons you give for not eating well (or for eating a bit too well!), not exercising, and not taking the time to slow down some, but it's time to begin living in alignment with your beliefs. We're not just totally spiritual beings—we've got a body housing that spirit. What can you do today to begin some "housecleaning?"

A Coaching Moment

Have you been trashing your temple? What do you need to do to start showing your body—and its Creator—the respect each deserves?

Stepping Stones

- Old baggage will only slow you down in your journey to wellness.
- Behavioral changes require four basic steps: desire, choice, planning, and action.
- Accepting cognitive or spiritual concepts ultimately boils down to one thing: a choice.

CHAPTER FOUR

Head Games, Body Games and Other Games Where No One Wins

Afew years back a friend and myself sat, sunk into big ol' comfy armchairs, chatting and catching up, teacups in hand. Like most conversations between two female friends, the topic of weight eventually came up. My friend, an Italian beauty, had struggled with her weight for as long as I had known her. "You know," she said. "I really wonder if there isn't something about having girls that makes the mother gain more weight." She, a mother of four girls, and myself, a mother of four boys, would have been perfect specimens for a research study on the topic. Of course, being a professional in the fitness field, I had to come up with something that sounded semi-scientific and intelligent, so after considering her statement for a moment, I answered, "Hmmm. That's a good question. Maybe it's something to do with all those extra female hormones you carry around for nine months—times four!" Well, it sounded good to me (and believe me–I'm not one who thinks off-the-cuff well at all!). And I think it made her feel better at the time, having been given a possible reason for the extra pounds (an albeit not-scientifically-proven-reason!). But haven't we all done that at some point? We play these games, hoping to trick ourselves into thinking that there really is a reason why we have the body we have. We carry on the blame game, blaming ourselves for having no willpower; blaming the images we see on T.V., in the movies, on magazine covers; blaming manufacturers for making the garbage that we have no willpower not to eat—and many, as we know, have even tried to benefit monetarily from that one! No doubt, some responsibility goes to the media for pushing unrealistic, fake images. And there is the whole pregnancy thing. Then there's the infamous slowing metabolism as we age. And while we're on a roll, who's really got the time to workout anyway?

A Coaching Moment

Who have you been blaming for your lack of success in making healthy changes? Is it truly the "others'" faults? Or is it really that you have been allowing them to influence you?

The Game of Perfection

"Pop! Goes Perfection!" Remember that game? Yep. Perfection is big business—and one of my personal pet peeves. How many magazine covers and ads do you see with titles like *"Fitness Rx: Your Ultimate Prescription for the Perfect Body?"* What does it take to achieve the perfect body? What about books? *There's Perfectly Fit, Sculpting Her Body Perfect, The Body Sculpting Bible for Women: The Way to Physical Perfection,* and *BodyFitness for Women: Your Way to Physical Perfection.* Blech. Believe me, I know that the title can sell the book—it's probably one of the reasons you picked up this book. But enough with the perfect theme! What is the perfect body anyway? I suppose if we could go back in time to the Garden of Eden (harp and a little theater smoke, please…) and take a peek at Eve we might know. But since that's an impossibility, we seem to be left to the creative imaginations of photo manipulators and plastic surgeons. What about the perfect fitness level? Personally, I haven't seen any recent studies on this one. You see they hook you into believing that you will look like the fitness models in their books or their magazines. It's like the proverbial dangling carrot. The problem is, even if you worked out as much as the women between the pages, you may not ever look like them. You will look like you. A fit you, but still you.

It's all a part of the head games the media plays with us, and it goes back to making us believe that we can have what they sell—usually perfection. But

> "Aim for success, not perfection. Never give up your right to be wrong, because then you will lose the ability to learn new things and move forward with your life. Remember that fear always lurks behind perfectionism. Confronting your fears and allowing yourself the right to be human can, paradoxically, make yourself a happier and more productive person." — *Dr. David M. Burns*

as we discussed previously, most of it is literally make-believe. They're saying, "Look. You can have these results, this body that you see right here, if you do what we say." But the photo isn't even real. So isn't that false advertising? Other companies get taken to court for such things. And yet we continue to put up with—and support, although sometimes unknowingly— false images on the covers of magazines.

"Lose a dress size in three days" the headline says. Turn the page and you'll find the latest tempting recipes. Low fat? Some, but more likely fat-laden and a far cry from even being considered healthy. Is it wrong to eat these foods? Of course not. But does it make sense to tell readers on one page how to diet their way to "thindomhood," and on the very next page tempt them with all kinds of delectable, mouth-watering treats? For some magazines, this is their goldmine. I suppose they hope that readers will try the recipes and then feel the need to diet. This vicious cycle retains buyers for their publication.

How about reading an article about eating disorders, and on the opposite page is an anorexic-looking model forcing a glossy-page smile in an attempt to sell you the latest, must-have product. Head games.

Then there are the countless headlines that read, "The Three BEST Exercises to Squeeze Away Your Inner Thighs, Rip Up Your Abs, and Give Your Butt and Bust a Boost." You take their advice to heart but to no avail. After the six-weeks-promised-results deadline passes and you still don't look like their poster girls, you wonder what you've done wrong. Probably nothing. As with most things in life, there is no one best way to do anything. It all depends on the individual. Chances are you've noticed some changes, maybe even incredible changes. But you are you, and you will have your own individual changes. What I find especially worth a chuckle is that one month they'll have the best arm exercises, and six months later, they'll have the same exact title but with a whole new set of exercises. So…which ones are the best?

But the media isn't all to blame. Quite frankly, much of the blame should be placed squarely on our own shoulders. As women, we have allowed the media to play the part they have. How? Mainly by buying their publications. By watching their shows. By buying their products. We even subscribe to long-time commitments of a publication. Then, each month we can go to our mailboxes and torture ourselves with the images between the pages. If it makes you feel bad about yourself, stop buying it! Don't dawdle at the magazine rack in the supermarket. Don't watch the fitness show where the women seem more interested in showing off their (manmade) cleavage than they do in instructing viewers on real fitness—and the men seem more interested in watching the women! Stop buying the products that seem more like an advertisement for sex than they do the product. Stop buying into the "secrets" of fitness or weight loss. There are no secrets to weight loss and fitness! "Latest developments," maybe, but no secrets.

A Coaching Moment

How do you feel the media has influenced you and how you feel about yourself? What products or publications do you currently support that make you feel bad about yourself? Will you continue to support them? If so, why? If not, how will you begin today to make this change?

As a writer, I often hear other writers complaining about editors and publications—mostly about wages and rights. Their gripe is usually something like, "They wouldn't even have their publication if it weren't for the writers!" This is true. The writers help create a product to sell. However, the flip side is that they also wouldn't have a publication if it weren't for the buyers! This is a big reason some publications go under. If it can't keep a large circulation of readers, it can't sell ads and products, and thus ceases to exist.

The irony in this is that the cover truly does sell the magazine. Statistics show that when a thin, beautiful woman is placed on the cover, it sells more magazines. In this demand-driven business, it's no wonder that editors, publishers, art directors, advertisers, and fashion designers think they are just giving us what we want. Business is business, and they need to make money to stay in it. It is obviously working—at least in the U.S. Both Australian and South African publishers claim they have used more normal-sized women for years, and say they are far ahead of the rest of the world in this respect. And after much urging from physicians and eating-disorders specialists and attending a body-image summit in 2000, British editors discovered just how much of the population suffers from eating disorders in the U.K. and the media's potential influence on this very problem. Following the summit, they agreed to begin using models who varied in shape and size.

Unfortunately, Americans seem light years behind. How many magazines do you see that really cater to normal, average, everyday women? Even many of the fitness magazines tend to promote an unrealistic image. As we already know, they tweak and trim, airbrush and enhance the photos. And the models they use either a.) are stick thin, b.) have mounds of bulging, manly, testosterone and steroid-induced androgynous bodies, c.) are world-class, professional athletes, or d.) are full-time fitness models. Which mold would you like to squeeze yourself into? As one editor puts it, "We're selling a dream." We all need dreams, goals, and aspirations, but you need to ask yourself if it's realistic and reachable for you, and whether or not the end result is worth your investment.

A Coaching Moment

Is your dream realistic for you? If not, how long are you going to chase an unattainable dream? How long are you going to base your life around the chase? Is the cost worth the investment?

Games (Other) People Play

Healthy-living saboteurs can be very good at playing head games with us. They come in all shapes, sizes, and relations— and sometimes are those we least expect. Whether it's done intentionally or not, the end result is the same: frustration.

In a recent *ivillage.com* article, Kathleen Zelman, R.D. a registered dietician and spokesperson for the American Dietetic Association (ADA), says there are several types of saboteurs when it comes to making healthy changes. First on the list is the "supportive spouse," who, while he says he supports your dedication to live healthier, doesn't necessarily show it by his actions. For instance, he brings home all the junk food he knows you love, and scarfs it down in front of you, incoherently mumbling in between bites, "I'd offer you some, but I know you're on a diet." Or he just happens to schedule a golf date with his buddies for the same night he knows you're planning on attending your first kickboxing class. When approached with the reminder that he had promised to watch the kids, he relents, "How hard can it be to find a babysitter?" In which case you should promptly hand over the phone and let him find out!

> "My favorite sabotage line is 'just this once,'" says Leanne Ely of Los Angeles, California. "Others do it to me, I do it to me...the fact is too many 'just this once' indulgences have me needing to take off about 25 pounds now!"

Then there's the "motherer" who tries to coerce you with the old, "C'mon! Just one more bite isn't going to hurt you,"

41

while practically force-feeding the other half of a double chocolate caramel nut cheesecake down your throat. The "motherer" can be one of the most threatening saboteurs, says Zelman, because she tends to be argumentative and counts on wearing you down to do what she says. She can also try to make you feel like you're making a big deal out of nothing, especially when she uses the "just this once" line.

If you work outside your home, you know all too well about your "junk-loving co-workers." From jelly doughnuts, to help chase away the manic-Monday blues to mid-week "Hump-Day" chocolate feasts, to pre-happy hour celebrations every Friday, the office can be a health-lover's worst nightmare. You plan on walking during your lunch hour, but they beg you to go out with them for lunch at the new pizza joint—"just this once." Throw in a "watchdog," someone who's keeping track of every morsel that passes your lips, and you've got a good defense for your insanity plea.

Carrie Rivera knows all about the head games other people can play. Perhaps the most frustrating thing is that they're not even consistent about it—unless you consider consistent inconsistency being consistent! And as Rivera found out, one person can be many different kinds of saboteurs all rolled into one.

"Although I thought growing up that I had a weight problem, reality struck when I hit 20 and became ill. Then the real weight problems began," explains Rivera. "The worst are the people who used to be really jealous of me and now really like me, but begin to act strangely when I start to show progress. Or, certain people who used to test me and 'tsk tsk' every time I chose to enjoy a dessert (watchdogs), now offer to bake, buy, or take me out for dessert (motherers). If I go they say, 'See, you're not being serious [about making healthy changes] (watchdogs), and if I don't go it's, 'You're being ridiculous' (motherers)."

Why people play these games can be pretty obvious. Can you say "little green monster?" We'd probably all be lying if we didn't admit that at one time or another we were jealous of another woman's ability to change. It's human nature. I mean, why do we go through the agony of subsisting on just fat free broth and celery sticks for two months before our high school reunion? Two reasons: one, to make, to all the jocks who either wouldn't give us the time of day or who broke our hearts, a little jab of the knife (eat your hearts out fellas!), and two, to make all the cheerleaders feel the same way! Yep. Jealousy can be a terrific motivator, especially when you're on the receiving end of it. But bring warm fuzzy feelings it doesn't. It can also be detrimental—detrimental to relationships, and detrimental to yourself.

Why people become jealous has different foundations. They may see you as a threat in some way, whether relationship-wise or even job-wise. Becoming more fit and confident may make you more attractive to the boss, who's looking for someone to give that new promotion to. They may already be jealous of you for other reasons—you have a great marriage and they don't, you have a beautiful house, they don't, whatever—and you becoming healthy and fit just adds to the already bountiful amounts of green stuff that oozes out of every nook and cranny. They could also be jealous that you've gone beyond just wanting to become healthier and are actually doing something about it. Of course, this is no foundation for jealousy (what is?), since everyone has the opportunity to choose to be as healthy as they can be—but they don't see it that way, because they're still tripping over their own excuses.

The "supportive husband" may be showing you he's a little insecure—especially if he's got a spare tire or two hanging around. Your determination to live a healthier lifestyle will most likely lead to a fitter, happier you, which in turn, in his mind, means attracting the wandering eyes of other men. And who knows where that will lead to! With the new you, will you still be happy with him?

Rather than getting angry at him for what he's doing, or giving up and joining him in all of his "feast fests," try being open and honest with him. Let him know how you feel. When a friend of mine had problems with her whole family being unsupportive of her changes, she sat down and talked to them about it. "I felt like every time I finally made the decision to make these changes, especially pertaining to exercise, my family took that as a cue to be even more demanding of my time."

Because of this, she found it extremely difficult to even begin, let alone stick with, an exercise program. Sitting down with her family and explaining how important it was to her to take better care of herself helped tremendously.

"Since doing that, I haven't had nearly as many obstacles to getting out for my walks."

Don't be afraid to invite your family to join you on your journey to health. Working as a team can make it easier, as long as you don't compare your progress to theirs. Your goal should be to be as healthy as *you* can be, regardless of where anyone else is on their journey.

"I just want you to be happy," retorts the "motherer." And it's true—in a sort of twisted, controlling way. If you've ever watched "Everybody Loves Raymond," you know what I mean. Perhaps you've lived with a "Marie," Ray's mother on the show. She truly does want Raymond to be happy—as long as she has a say in how it's done. With "motherers" the main crux of finding this happiness is through food—often, food they've made for you. By you eating what they make, it's like saying, "I accept you." By showing that you like what they bake, it's like you're saying, "I love you." It's the guilt trap, because if you don't eat, you feel guilty. If you do eat it you feel just as guilty. You Italian girls know what I'm talking about! "Mangiare! Mangiare!" And if you don't "mangiare!", feelings are hurt, and you probably end up eating anyway—extra helpings to make up for it, and so the guilt compounds. As with the "supportive husband," honesty is the best policy when dealing with a "motherer." Explain that you love her for who she is. Tell her how much you enjoy her food and appreciate her kindness and effort, but that you're trying to take better care of yourself, which includes making some healthier choices—like eating when you're hungry, not just because someone else wants you to eat. You might also want to mention that the human stomach was just not designed to hold that much food!

> For Lynn Shaw, MSW, a "plus-size" fitness professional and creator of Laugh-A-Size™, the bottom line when making healthy changes is support. "I surround myself with people who are truthful and caring. I have several girlfriends who support me in whatever phase of my journey I am traveling. I am becoming more honest about my self-assessment and am sharing more openly about my plans, flaws, successes, etc. It can be quite freeing."

So what do you do if the saboteurs in your life don't listen? In the words of Carrie Rivera, "get rid of the people who are destructive and set straight the ones you can't get rid of."

Whoa! Pretty tough, huh? But as the old saying goes, "You can pick your friends, you can pick your nose, but you can't pick your family." (This is the type of wisdom I glean from raising a house full of boys!) To some extent—okay, a lot of extent—we have control over who we hang out with. If someone is bringing you down, and you've tried to be honest and deal with their sabotaging efforts, it may be time to separate yourself from them—at least for a while.

"I realized that I was killing myself to make other people feel better. I had traded health for friendship, which, of course, wasn't really friendship. Rather than trust in God and respect myself, I tried to deal with it all myself. I did a major housecleaning of people and I am sad, but I'm getting a clearer idea of the life I want and will have."

> "No one can make you feel inferior without your consent."
> —Eleanor Roosevelt

It works in reverse, too. Try encircling yourself with people who are encouraging, truthful, and aren't out for just themselves.

A Coaching Moment

Who are the healthy-living saboteurs in your life? What category do they fall under: motherer, watchdog, green monster, just-once sayers, or "supportive husbands?" What do you need to do today to stop their influence?

Head Games, Starring...You!

Like I said before, not all the responsibility can or should be placed on others. It begins with us. Not only do we tend to allow others to play games with us, but we also play them with ourselves. When I became anorexic while in high school, it started with head games. First (aside from the underlying psychological issues), there's the whole distorted body image thing where I convinced myself that I was fat. Compared to what I saw in the media, I guess I had good reason to believe this. But realistically, I was average. Then there's the thinking that if I could just become thinner, I'd be loved more. It's a head game having to do with taking the truth—I am loved as I am—and twisting it—I'll be loved more based on my external appearance.

Most of us play head games to some extent. For Kawon Lee, mother of three, it's taking real possibilities and exaggerating them into current reality. "As I start to plan out my daily schedule for the next few months in an effort to lose weight, I literally see everything unraveling right in front of my eyes. The house might get on fire because the nanny forgot to turn off the stove. Then the kids will have to be rescued by fire fighters. If that doesn't happen they will hurt themselves playing and will have to be rushed to the hospital but the nanny doesn't drive. If that doesn't happen they will open the door for some stranger who turns out to be a burglar. While all this is going on in my mind, I have laid the keys down and am in the middle of fixing a snack because I have convinced myself that being fat is better than being in misery for an hour-and-a-half at the gym everyday wondering what tragedy has befallen the children."

I had to laugh when I read Kawon's statement, because I've done the exact same thing (minus the nanny part!). We might be in an accident on the way to the gym and all die, or if we do make it to the gym, some abductor (that's the child one, not the muscle!) might come and steal the kids out of the nursery. After our club added a pool, the excuse was my little one might escape out of the nursery and end up in the pool and no one will know he's there and he'll drown.

Sometimes these fears are based on something real that has happened in the past. In Kawon's case, her son actually was hurt once while she was gone. For others, it's the "what if" syndrome. What if someone is hurt while I'm gone? What if we're in an accident on the way there? What if someone takes the kids? Obviously, this can be a sign of a more serious anxiety disorder, in which case, help should be sought. But for many, it's allowing our imaginations and fears to get the best of us—and one more reason to find an excuse not to change.

Another reason for this head game was also voiced directly by Kawon when she said, "being fat is better..." Fat can be comforting. Fat can be a safety net. Fat can be a shield from the outside world, especially when you feel vulnerable. Being fat means being able to sink into the surroundings without being noticed. You can melt into the background and nobody sees you.

Carrie Rivera relates to this. A former child model, Carrie has born the brunt of other women's jealousy all her life. She has also attracted a lot of inappropriate behavior from men she refers to as creeps. "I traded muscles and beauty—which didn't keep me safe—for a fat, unattractive body."

After being in the spotlight during her modeling days, Carrie fell ill and gained weight. "It was extremely comfortable being fat. Girlfriends felt very comfortable introducing me to their significant others. My husband didn't have to have his guard up every time we went out, as other men would hit on me. I didn't have problems at work with being hit on or jealousy and I felt like I could go anywhere because no one pays attention to the fat girl."

A Coaching Moment
How do you tend to sabotage your own efforts? Are the reasons you give really excuses in disguise?

Numbers, Numbers Everywhere

For many of us, the scale has been the basis of our head games. If we've got a doctor's appointment scheduled, we won't eat all day. I mean everyone knows how many ounces a salad and a glass of water add to the scale. We've made sure to wear the lightest underwear, even if it means the annoyance of a day-long thong wedgie. Shoes? Gone! We remove every last piece of jewelry on us, except for the wedding rings that we swore would never come off—nope, them, too! We do some quick, fidgety movements and throw in a bicep contraction or two in the hopes of knocking off a few last minute calories.

"The scale is my favorite weapon of choice," laughs Shirley Kawa-Jump. "For instance, when I step on the scale, I let out all my breath, even though I know the weight of air is nil. I feel

> If we've got balance in our habits, there is no need for reward or punishment. Instead, it all just becomes a part of our lives.

lighter then. If I'm up a bit, I blame it on that cup of coffee or the salt on my dinner last night. If I don't see the weight I want to see on the readout, I'll weigh myself a couple more times during the day until it comes back down. If it doesn't, then I'm eating salad for lunch and vowing to diet. That lasts about a day. Then, if I know I'm eating poorly, I'll avoid the scale instead, shoving it into the closet so I don't have that reminder that I'm not sticking to the program."

Ah, yes. The Program. And if we don't stick to it, we don't deserve…what? And if we do stick to it, then by all means, we deserve a reward, right?

"I always tell myself that I have earned that piece of chocolate, that glass of wine, the entire Sarah Lee® cheesecake," laughs one woman.

We seem to need a reason to enjoy simple pleasures—even necessary ones, like eating. This probably stems from childhood when our mothers said things like, "If you behave today, we can go out for supper tonight" or "If you eat everything on your plate (read: eat it whether you like it or not and whether or not you're hungry) you can have dessert." Using food as a basis for reward and punishment is not a good idea. It's also hard not to do it! Now, I'm not referring to the occasional reward—you've met a huge goal or deadline and want to reward yourself with lobster or a night out to your favorite restaurant, for instance. I'm talking about the daily rewards and punishments we place upon ourselves. "I had a hard day and deserve this package of cookies." "My best friend totally blew me off. I must have done something to upset her. I need this pizza—all of it!" One thing you must get straight in your own mind and come to the point of accepting, is that no food (no matter how much chocolate it contains!) will bring you emotional peace. That piece of cheesecake will not decrease your stress. Stuffing a box of donuts down your throat will not take the pain of losing a loved one away. Super-sizing your fries will not reconcile lost love. Whether you're justifying these behaviors in your mind by saying, "I deserve this" (reward) or by saying, "I'm no good, so what's the use" (punishment) or even by thinking, "I don't deserve that" (punishment by withholding), you will not feel better by doing any of these actions. In fact, this type of attitude and behavior will only perpetuate the whole self-loathing cycle.

A Coaching Moment

In what ways do you reward or punish yourself with food? What emotions trigger unhealthy eating? Keep a food journal and track what you eat, when you eat it, and what emotions you're feeling at the time. Boredom counts, too!

By recognizing what emotions trigger emotional eating, you can then find other, healthier, more fulfilling behaviors to engage in during those times. By not making a list of forbidden foods—those foods you aren't allowed to eat—you can include all foods, in moderation and balance, into your plan. This type of balance negates the cycle of using food as reward and punishment. If we've got balance in our habits, there is no need for reward or punishment. Instead, it all just becomes a part of our lives.

A Coaching Moment

What are some ways you can begin incorporating balance into your life so that punishing yourself is no longer necessary?

51

Tomorrow, Tomorrow...

"Tomorrow, tomorrow, I love ya, tomorrow..." As an Annie wannabe, I used to belt out that tune when I was a little girl. And while its lyrics give hope that better days are coming, we can use it as an excuse to keep putting a healthier, more nurturing lifestyle on hold.

"One head game I play with myself is promising 'tomorrow' things will be different," says Leanne Ely. "Tomorrow I will exercise, tomorrow I'll drink more water."

Ely, herself a nutritionist, knows how difficult it can be to give up the head games, even when you have the knowledge to do otherwise. "It's easy to justify and rationalize anything if you're skilled enough!" she laughs. "I know for me, I will not eat healthy or exercise because I've not taken the time to schedule it. I have to schedule everything or nothing gets done."

Every choice has a "pay-off," as well, adds Ely. And while at the time, the pay-off may seem like it pays positive dividends, in the long run, you end up in the red. "When I make an unhealthy choice, the pay-off at the time is that I've 'saved' time—by driving through the drive-thru, for instance. But in the end, all I feel is lousy—not to mention it's done nothing for my body. So while the benefits are sometimes perceived as benefits for the moment, in the long run, they end up as detriments."

Tricky!

Another head game that appears to be quite popular is one that involves tricking yourself into believing that certain foods don't appeal to you any more.

"I began to tell myself that I didn't like the taste of certain foods, trying to fool myself into not eating them," explains one young woman. "The one item that sticks in my mind is butter. I successfully convinced myself that I hated butter until one day a roommate put butter on some toast and I had a bite. I realized that for nearly five years I had been playing a game with myself, and butter didn't taste all that bad, especially in moderation."

This is the head game that helped me control what I ate when I was anorexic. I, too, would tell myself that I didn't like certain foods. Or I would think, "You can have that anytime, why have it now?" The whole irony is that this can be used as a tool to stop playing this head game, and actually make some healthy changes, because it can help distinguish between eating due to hunger and emotional eating.

Sharon Anne Waldorp says that when she's noticed a few-pound weight gain she can take it off easily by reminding herself "food is simply a means of survival, and not a nurturing tool or entertainment item. If I remind myself to eat just enough healthy foods to make it through the day—and trust me, I have to remind myself of this out loud and often—I can shed the extra pounds that creep on my body. So when I'm looking at a piece of boysenberry pie and saying out loud for everyone to hear, 'I need food to survive, but I don't need that piece of boysenberry pie,' it's easy to walk away from it."

A Coaching Moment

What tricks do you use to fool yourself into thinking that you're healthier than you are? Do you try to trick yourself into thinking you don't need some form of food?

When this mind set is taken to extremes, however, it can become dangerous, as in my case. I took the "means to survival" and pushed it to its limits. If you've ever watched the show "Survivor," you know that during those 40 days in the wilderness, the participants eat minimally. This is eating to survive. But they suffer some consequences. Lack of proper nutrition quickly takes its toll on a body, mind, and spirit. When we go the route of using food simply as a means to survive, we miss out on eating to thrive and the joy that can be derived by it. As women, we seem to feel guilty for liking food, for actually enjoying a good meal. I've read several times in various magazines throughout the years that men love it when they take a woman on a date and she actually eats! Single men are so used to taking women out on dates and having them pick at a salad while he chows down a Porter House, that it's nice when she actually enjoys the meal. This isn't to say that we should pig out every time we eat. The point I'm trying to get across is that it's okay to enjoy what you're eating, whether it's a ripe, juicy peach, a

> If you're not enjoying what's on the end of your fork then drop it, put your hands in the air, and slowly step away from the table!

grilled chicken breast, or that Sara Lee® cheesecake. It's all about balance.

It's also about making a distinction between using food as nourishment and using it as nurturance. This is tricky, because the two root words nourish and nurture, both come from similar original Latin roots, which means "to suckle." And what do infants get when they suckle? Food. But they also receive nurturing during the actual feeding. Is it the food that causes them to be nurtured…or the environment—the closeness to their mother's breast and body, the warmth, love, and closeness they feel, the feeling of safety? Perhaps a little bit of each. The food is soothing their grumbly tummies, making them feel better physically. The environment is also meeting their needs—physically, mentally, and emotionally. Studies show that infants who do not receive physical touch, do not develop properly. Regardless of the fact that they're being fed, they can be physically smaller, emotionally underdeveloped, have very poor motor skills, and even exhibit behaviors similar to autism.

How does this apply to you? By trying to fill some void with food, you do nothing but fill the void between your muscles and skin! Just as food cannot meet the emotional needs of infants, it cannot meet yours. Using food to nurture your spirit, heal past hurts and pains, and to fill voids only leads to compulsive, comfort, emotional eating—which in the end does nothing but create more pain and a larger waistline.

> "Food and love. We begin eating compulsively because of reasons that have to do with the kind and amount of love that is in our lives or that is missing from our lives. If we haven't been loved well, recognized, understood, we arrange ourselves to fit the shape of our situations. We lower our expectations. We stop asking for what we need. We stop showing the places that hurt or need comfort. We stop expecting to be met. And we begin to rely on ourselves and only ourselves to provide sustenance, comfort, and pleasure. We begin to eat. And eat." Excerpted from *When Food is Love: Exploring the Relationship Between Eating and Intimacy,* by Geneen Roth, Plume - 1992

It can work the other way around, too, as in the case of anorexia. Rather than eating to heal, we don't eat, to heal. In an attempt to gain control over the pain, we withhold food, proving that we are stronger than the pain. Bulimics shove food down their throats in an attempt to bury their feelings and hurt, but then panic and purge, offering a temporary panacea. But in the end, no matter which method is chosen, the end result is just more pain and guilt. I'm living proof, however, that you can end the cycle! You can stop playing head games with yourself and you can stop allowing others to influence your decisions about yourself. And you hold the keys: desire, choose, plan, and act!

Stepping Stones

- While others try to sabotage our efforts, we are often to blame for allowing them to do so.
- If it makes you feel bad about yourself, don't buy it!
- Head games are things we do to ourselves or that others do to us to alter our state of reality.
- You'll never move ahead in your journey if you continue to play the blame game.

CHAPTER FIVE

Sizing It All Up

One of the first bridges many women must cross in their journey is that of acceptance. Size acceptance, body acceptance, self-acceptance—each one is a stepping stone to a much larger issue. You must possess size acceptance before you can move on to body acceptance. You must have body acceptance before you can be fully self-accepting. Why? Because each one is a part of the next. Let's take a look at each one more carefully.

Size Acceptance— Owning Up, Getting On

Women's sizes are an enigma, aren't they? I mean, at 5'4"—okay, okay (for all of you who know me), it's just a smidgen under 5'4"—average weight and build for my height, I can wear a range of three different sizes. It depends on the cut, style, and brand of the clothing. Because of this variance, I gave up the notion a long time ago that I had to fit into a certain size. I choose my clothing based on comfort as much as I do on style. If that means buying the larger size, so be it. Of course, this wasn't always the case. While anorexic, I could wear a size 0 (one of my twisted goals!). But I'm here to say, it didn't make me any happier—and it certainly didn't make me healthier.

As women, we tend to get really hung up on what size we are. I suppose stores don't help us out in this area, since they totally separate the "plus" sizes from "normal" sizes. And let's face it, many of the plus-size sections more closely resemble the camping section than they do a clothing department. Manufacturers have even come up with feminine protection for plus-sized women—as if they have larger vaginas or something.

Because we hesitate to be labeled plus-sized, a more inferior human species, we dare not cross that threshold into the black hole in the small corner of the store, afraid we may never come back to "normalness." So we continue to squeeze ourselves into clothing that should have been given away during the Reagan era. Do you fit into this category? If you're unsure, a good indicator is this: if, by the end of the day (sooner for some), you can no longer feel your legs due to the circulation being cut off by your waistband, take my word— you do belong here.

On the other hand, some women have grown very comfortable with their plus-sizeness. This is okay if they're choosing growth along with it—and I don't mean girth size. While I applaud the "fat acceptance" movement for their mission in attempting to stamp out fat phobia and stereotypes, I also feel it has muddied the waters a bit on self-nurturance, self-growth, and self-improvement, and trying to get women moving towards being the best and healthiest they can be. I remember once seeing a show where a very beautiful, seemingly very happy fat woman, who had accepted her fate in life, was cooking up a colossal breakfast of bacon, sausage, and eggs—the real deal—and I wondered if her intestines, heart, and arteries were as happy as she appeared to outwardly be with what they were being fed.

I'm not the one to judge, of course, but it seems this type of woman has surrendered to her size. I know you're thinking that I'm preaching a double message here. I mean, after all, isn't this book on loving yourself no matter where you are in life? No matter what size you are? And shouldn't you accept your God-given size? Yes. But there is a very fine line separating accepting your size and surrendering to it.

Surrendering to your size means you have accepted the size you currently inhabit, and that is all. You no longer strive for a better you. You don't bother to ask yourself if this is your true size—the size you are really meant to be. You have grown so "comfortable" with where you're at now, that you have given up on nurturing the person inside the size. This is not true size acceptance. This, in effect, is self-loathing, because you are no longer providing yourself with what you need to be the best person you could be. You've sunk yourself into this big, over-sized couch, unwilling to budge from it.

Truly accepting your size also involves accepting your current size. Those of you who need to check a mirror to make sure your lower body still exists (because in the time it took you to read this section so far, you've lost circulation and your legs are numb) need to admit and accept what your current size really is. Be honest with yourself. Stop squeezing into those size 10 pants, when you'd be much more comfortable in a size 12 or 14. This doesn't give you license, however, to become a slob. I know it can be difficult to find neat, stylish clothes at the plus-size level, but they are out there. Find them. Get some outfits that actually fit, and throw out or give away the ones that don't—all of them. Even the ones hiding in the back of your closet, or stored away in some bag or trunk up in the attic, awaiting the day you can fit back into them. Get rid of them.

Their main purpose is in taunting you, teasing you, giving you one more excuse to feel bad about yourself. Admit the size you're currently at. Accept it—then move on.

A Coaching Moment

What is your real, current size? Have you been squeezing into an unrealistic size? It's time to get real! What do you need to do to fill your wardrobe with clothes that fit?

But, you ask, if I should strive for the best I can be, why get rid of those old clothes? Isn't that what I should be striving for? Excellent question! Be sure to not equate a size—or for that matter, a number on the scale,

> Size acceptance is as much about moving on as it is accepting where you're currently at.

either—with being well. Nor should you strive for a certain size. Instead, strive for a state of well-being. All these years you've been trying to attain a smaller size. Sometimes you reach it, at which time, the clothes come out from hiding. But then the weight creeps back, and back go the "thin" clothes, out come the "fat" ones. Holding onto and labeling all these clothes gives you an excuse to concentrate on your weight and unhealthy measures for attaining what some chart says you should weigh, rather than striving to live in wellness, no matter what your current size. When you live a life of wellness and you're taking care of yourself in all areas of your life the best you can, your body will find its true size. As you begin your journey and your body begins to re-regulate itself, get rid of the clothes that are too big and baggy and get ones that fit (again). Stashing away the larger clothes—just in case—can be too much of a security blanket. It gives you an excuse to go back to old habits and not take care of yourself, so get rid of them!

After admitting and owning up to your current size, it's time to ask yourself what your true size is. This is the major differing factor between size acceptance and size surrendering. In size surrendering, you don't move on. You accept your "fate," and think of it as some sort of life sentence. Size acceptance is as much about moving on as it is accepting where you're currently at.

Your true size is the size your body is happy being at. This works from both ends of the spectrum. Are you starving yourself or obsessively working out or taking drugs or purging to try to maintain a certain weight or size? If you have to do excessive, unnatural things to try to keep your weight down, you're not at your true size! Many former "skinny-turned-plus-size" models came to this realization.

Coming from the other end, if you've been using one excuse after another as to why you eat the way you do and why you don't exercise and why you don't take care of yourself, there's a good chance you're also not at your true size. By making the choice to take care of yourself and give yourself what you need to be well, you will find your true size.

Once you've accepted and owned up to your current size, and you've begun to make the changes necessary to discover your true size, you've made that first step toward a larger issue: body acceptance.

A Coaching Moment

Have you ever been at your true size? If so, how did you feel at that time? Did you feel good? How are your habits different now than they were back then?

Stop Tearing Yourself Apart!

Body acceptance and body image are both terms that have been thrown into the spotlight with the emergence of our modern-day eating disorders. What is the difference between the two? Body image is how you see your body—your physical image. When you look into the mirror, what do you see? When an anorexic sees her image, although she's often skin and bones, she "sees" fat. This is a distorted image. Most of us, however, see our image for what it is. Whether or not we accept it is another thing…and herein lies the difference. Body acceptance is about taking the image we see and accepting it for what it is—being real about it. Like size acceptance, body acceptance is also about moving on, while at the same time accepting the big picture. What can you reasonably and realistically change about your body? What can't you? What genes has heredity dealt you? What is your natural body shape? Are you curvaceous and womanly? Are you straight up and down? Are you an apple or a pear—big on top, small on bottom—or visa versa? What is the size of your skeleton? What is your normal level of hormones, like testosterone (it's not just for men!), which partly determines how much muscle you'll have, which in turn helps regulate your metabolism? What about your personal history? Were you an overweight child? If so, you probably have more fat cells inside your body, whether you were born with them or your body more readily produced them due to your lifestyle and eating habits.

Scientists have construed varying fat-cell theories about whether or not we actually add fat cells—or are we born with what we've got and will never have more or less—just

> While we need to accept our limitations, we also cannot use them as an excuse to not take care of ourselves.

full or empty cells? It's the old hypertrophy v. hyperplasia debate. Are we born with all the fat cells we'll ever have, and they just get bigger and bigger as more fat is stored? Or do our bodies actually produce more fat cells as the demand for them (as we ingest more calories than we're using) increases (the whole supply and demand thing)? It appears that it's a little bit of both—our fat cells do fluctuate between full and empty, and there are probably times in our lives when we can actually add fat cells: during the third trimester in utero, the first two years of life, and during the post-puberty period. Some researchers are also investigating the theory that some women's metabolisms slow down following pregnancy. This may help explain many women's age-old complaint about the post-pregnancy body and how it's never the same again. However, many of us don't help ourselves in this respect, either. The stick turns blue and we suddenly have been handed a license to eat anything and everything. Exercise? Why? We use pregnancy as our excuse to avoid healthy habits, when in reality, it should be our number one reason to indulge in such things.

My whole point here is two-fold: while we need to accept our limitations, we also cannot use them as an excuse to not take care of ourselves. It's back to the surrender v. acceptance thing. Be realistic about your body. Is it reasonable for you to want Cindy Crawford's body when you're 5'2," large-framed, and stout? Of course not!

We can mess around with certain physiological aspects some, but only to a certain extent. And then you must ask yourself to what price? You could pop any number of pills to help increase your muscle mass or metabolism…or you could exercise and eat healthy foods. The question to ask yourself is, which is more nurturing? First of all, if you're just popping the pills (or mixing the shakes…), you're not taking time for you. It's more of the quick-fix mentality. It's that "hoping-for-a-magic-pill" thing. It's about not taking responsibility for yourself and nurturing your body. It's about using excuses for why you're in the shape you're in.

A Coaching Moment

Paint a word-portrait about your body. Use creative language to describe how you see your body. Then read it back to yourself. Do you focus on the negative aspects of it? If so, rework your masterpiece to give a more balanced view. Don't forget to include the marvelous functions your body performs for you.

Ask any woman what body part she'd change if she could, and she will immediately point out at least one "flaw" that has plagued her, her entire life. Most likely, however, she will fill you in on many parts! For me, it's always been this little roll in my lower abs. As far back as I can remember this has bothered me. I grew up with two very skinny cousins, who, to my naked eye, had no bodily flaws. I felt fat and inferior in this respect. My little "pooch" seemed to hang out all over the place. And a bathing suit? Forget it! I felt like a big blob next to them.

However, looking back at pictures, I realize what a distorted body image I had, even as a little girl. I was quite thin, with long, lean legs. Any sign of this potbelly sure doesn't show up in any photos I've got! But the feelings of dismay for this body part continued into adulthood. One reason I loved being pregnant was because for once in my life, I didn't have to worry about "the roll," and having to suck my gut in. I loved feeling the baby grow and move inside of me. And I loved my pregnant belly...until, that is, I gave birth. Then it reappeared—and it brought friends—lots and lots of saggy skin and stretch marks. My little nemesis was trying to ruin my life—and at a time when baring your midriff was just coming into vogue, too! Not to mention, as a fitness professional, it's quite well-known that a sign of "true fitness" is one mean looking six-pack—or in the very least, flat, almost concave abs. How many fitness videos do you not see participants bearing their abs? I can't think of too many. It really has become a symbol in our society of separating the truly fit from the not-so-truly fit. So this just added to my anxiety.

After four pregnancies, however (with the stretch marks moving further and further East, West, North, and South!), I knew I had to do some reconciling with my middle. I just could not continue to bemoan the fact that this body part had changed—and not for the better (and I thought just the little roll was bad?). I had to make a choice to stop coveting all those gorgeous abs on television, many of which are probably surgically enhanced anyway. Hey! These are my abs—stretch marks and all! I own them! My wonderful husband, I must admit, played a significant role in my "poochie recovery." He dubbed my stretch marks my "badges of honor," and said that he loves that part of my body, because it housed our four sons. (Awww...) I know. Sweet, huh?

Maybe your husband doesn't show the same kind of empathic regard, but you can still make the choice to accept whatever body part has been taunting you all these years. Maybe it's your hips or your thighs or your breasts. Whatever it is, love it, accept it, and nurture it. I nurture my abs by making them stronger and massaging them with moisturizer. Do they look like what you'll see in the latest fitness magazine? No. And they probably never will—unless they come up with some form of a home airbrushing unit. But I can still help them be the best abs they can be, without being obsessive about them.

When we tear ourselves apart, or nit pick little parts of us, or say, "If only I could get rid of..." we can't possibly come to a place of total body acceptance. Therefore, you'll never come to a place of self-acceptance, since your body is a part of you.

People who are obsessed with the belief that a certain body part is ugly or abnormally shaped are known to have body dysmorphic disorder or BDD. While the grand majority of us do not fall into this category, we tend to do the same thing as the BDDers do to themselves, just to a lesser extent. And the result can be nearly as damaging. When we see our bodies as parts and pieces rather than as a whole, we will almost always find something to be dissatisfied with. This part will be too big, that part will be too small, this other part will be too lumpy, and that part—well, we won't even go there! Stop treating yourself like you're buying cuts of meat at a grocery store!

A Coaching Moment

Is there a part of your body you would change if you could? What is it? What can you do to begin nurturing that part of your body?

How many times have you gone to a pool or the beach, refusing to get into a bathing suit? You sit there, baking to death in the scorching sun, thinking the whole time how inviting the water looks and how refreshing—and fun—it would be if you could just run and cannonball right into it (and how utterly surprised your friends would be!). You sigh as you mop the sweat from your brow and go back to reading your book. How many opportunities have you missed out on because you just "couldn't be seen wearing that?"

So What's a Girl To Do?

First of all, buy a new bathing suit that fits! Go someplace where you can try them on. I'm the first to admit that this can be an extremely anxious event, and ranks right up there with having a tooth pulled—without Novocain. In fact, I recently returned from just such an excursion. My husband could not understand why my mood went so quickly from "Yeah! A new bathing suit (and reason to go shopping!)" to "If only I could afford liposuction." It's not the easiest task. But it is possible.

A Coaching Moment

Is there an activity you used to enjoy or have been dying to try, but won't because of embarrassment over your body? In what ways do you put life on hold, simply because of what you look like?

Next, do what we all ready said about nurturing the areas of your body you don't like. Rather than hide them or pretend they're not there, look them straight in the eye and tell them that since they're not going anywhere, darn it, you're just going to accept them. However, things are going to change from here on out. From now on, you're going to give them the attention they need. You're going to take care of them and include them in your body as a whole.

Try celebrating your body as a whole and what it can do rather than just what it looks like. Maybe you've neglected taking care of your body all these years, however, so it doesn't even do what it should. That's okay, because that's something you can change. Have you ever given birth? That's quite a feat, wouldn't you say? What about breastfeeding? Remarkable! The human body is totally amazing. Think of all the intricate details that go on inside your body every second you're alive. Regardless of whether or not you could run a marathon right now, it's still an incredible machine, and one that deserves your attention and care.

Make a decision to take back your body and claim it as your own. Nurture it and take care of it as you would an infant. Would you allow a child to purposely go days without proper rest, nutrition, and cleanliness? Dr. Phil explained this very well one day on "Oprah" when he said something like this: pretend you are a life manager…and you are your only client. What advice would you be giving your client? Would you tell her it's okay to not take any time for herself and run herself ragged? Would you tell her it's okay to always put everyone else first? Would you tell her not to bother to shower or eat well or exercise? Of course not! Chances are, you've given a friend some very similar advice at some time. It's very easy to say all this, but it's a very different matter actually doing it. If you've got small children, it may mean finding a babysitter to watch them while you take time to go to the gym or out for a walk. It may mean getting your husband to stay with the kids while you go grocery shopping alone (okay, I have to admit that even this most arduous task is more enjoyable when I can go by myself!) It may mean being more assertive the next time your boss expects you to work late, simply because you're the single girl. (I mean, c'mon how much of a life can a single woman have?!) It may mean asking for someone else's help so that you can take the time to take care of yourself.

As women, we're givers and managers. But being in this position also places us in a very controlling role. When we're the ones always giving, we don't have to become vulnerable and depend on anyone else. In the process, we become martyrs. We can do it all! But can we do it all well?

A Coaching Moment

How is your bountiful giving actually masquerading a much deeper desire for control?

So, now we've seen how size acceptance moves us toward body acceptance. Are you getting it? Are you seeing how much wasted time and energy is spent on not taking care of yourself and wishing you could have or be something different? It's really a great contradiction. Our number one excuse for not taking care of ourselves is that we don't have the time. When in reality, we've got nothing but time! When you take care of yourself—body, mind, and spirit—the way you should, and live your life on purpose (we'll get to this one in a bit), you'll find you have enough time for everything you need to do.

Things fall into place, you're healthier, your family is healthier, and your time is better spent. More on this later. Now let's move on to total self-acceptance.

Total self-acceptance is all of you. It's the whole shebang, the total package, the big picture. It's taking who you are as a person—body, mind, and spirit—accepting it, and, as with size and body acceptance, moving forward from where you're at today, this moment. It's about not letting other people's opinions of you determine who you are. How many of us try to squeeze into that mold?

I'm not saying we should totally ignore others' criticisms of us—sometimes they will have valid points that we should consider—but we shouldn't let others define who we are. Remember our story about the Wemmicks? Do you let other people put stickers on you? Whether they're mostly golden star stickers or gray circle stickers, true self-acceptance and joy does not come from other people's applause or criticism.

I believe true self-acceptance comes from accepting God's love and knowing Him through His Son, Jesus. After all, God created us. Do you believe He made some sort of mistake when He created you? The Scriptures are really cool if you take the time to dig into them. In there, you'll see many examples of how God loves, knows, and takes care of you. It even says He knew you before you were conceived, and that He knit you in your mother's womb. It talks about how if he cares about a bird and making sure it gets what it needs, how much more He cares for us!

Where do you draw your self-esteem from? Work? Family? Your external beauty? Your belongings: house, car, clothing? The size of your bank statement? The number of friends you have? Having the "right" friends? Let's suppose for a moment, that all this was taken away from you. Pick your own scenario, but for now, let's choose a car accident—no, a burning car accident—in which you are the sole survivor from your immediate family. Your face is burnt beyond recognition, you lose your friends, because they can't deal with it, you lose your job, because you can't work due to the accident—and since you can't work, you also lose your house and many of your prized possessions, no longer being able to afford any of it. It's just little ol' you. Everything you depended on to give you worth and meaning is gone. You are in a sense, stripped bare. Now how do you feel about yourself? Where's your self-worth now? Chances are it's well on its way to the sewage plant.

A Coaching Moment

Draw a picture of yourself in the middle of the page—go ahead—decorate it and make it look like you! Now, all around you, write in those things you pull your self-worth from. Then cross everything out, but yourself. How do you feel about what's left?

While we may draw pleasure from the things we have, and consider many things in our lives to be important to us, we cannot draw our self-worth from them. If we do, and those things are taken away, what is left? You must feel as though you are worth taking care of, regardless of what you possess or who you have in your life. Don't get me wrong, I would be devastated to lose anyone in my family or to have my face melted off. There is a definite process of grief that anyone in that type of situation must go through to get to the point of healing. But ultimately, when we derive our self-esteem and worth from fleeting, temporal things, it's not real self-worth. We can't build a house on sand with no foundation and expect it to stand—and yet we do it with ourselves. The foundation must be a relationship with our Creator. That is the only way to get—and keep—any real self-worth.

Another part of self-worth also comes from making a choice to love ourselves for who we are and how He created us. This doesn't mean, however, that we are to be passive rag dolls, taking a back seat and expecting Him to give us whatever we want. We can pray all we want for good health, for instance, and He may or may not oblige. But shame on us for expecting good health when we don't even take care of one of the gifts He gave us—our bodies. Your body is a gift. Your mind is a gift. And your spirit is a gift. We tend to take all this for granted. We also tend to take better care of "stuff"—things that carry a price tag—than we do priceless items, like our bodies, minds, and spirits. How far will your car go when the gas gauge reads empty or the oil light reminds you you're out of oil? Not too far. I know some people (we'll pick on the men now!) who wash, wax, and vacuum their cars every weekend. They never go over the recommended mileage before changing the oil. You could eat off their engines. While they're doing all this, they've got a cigarette in one hand and beer number six in the other (and it's only 11 AM). Their guts hang over into tomorrow, and the last time they laid eyes on anything fitness-related was in last night's infomercial.

What's wrong with this picture? And how do we, as women, differ from this scenario? *But it's my body, mind, and spirit*, you say. *I can do what I want with them.* You're right. They are yours. But they're also God's—His gift to each of us—and He will take them back in His timing. Hmm. When you start to look at it like that—that our bodies, minds, and spirits are sort of "on loan" for this lifetime—it kind of puts it in a whole new light, doesn't it?

A Coaching Moment

Do you honestly believe that your body is yours to do with it as you please? If so, keep on keeping on! But if not, what do you need to start doing right now to take care of your very precious gift?

How do you take care of something you've borrowed from someone else? Do you throw it against the wall? Beat it down into the ground and stomp on it? Scratch it all up? I certainly hope not (and if you do, remind me to never let you borrow anything of mine!). Consider your body, mind, and spirit on loan from your Creator, and things that you'll have to give back someday. Accept His gifts and take care of them!

For those of you who aren't buying this perspective, let me put a different spin on it. You say that your body, mind, and spirit are yours, but it seems to me that many of us have given ourselves away to things like the media, other people's opinions, and manufacturers' products. We let the media and others label us and determine who we are and how we feel about ourselves. We use (or eat) products to try to look a certain way—the way society says we should look if we are to be of any value. We take every little hurtful thing people say and store it away and allow it to pound our self-esteem down further and further until it's practically non-existent

.

A Coaching Moment

Where are you in your journey toward self-acceptance? In what ways have you given yourself away to the media, products, or others' opinions? What do you need to do today to free yourself from this trap?

I've struggled with these things throughout my lifetime. Since I was a child, I've taken other people's painful words, and hidden them somewhere deep down inside of myself. For each word, a little piece of my self-esteem was chipped away. I also allowed the media to define who I should be and what I should look like, which acted like an ax to chop away at any self-esteem left. I gave myself away and for a while, even lost myself when I allowed anorexia to take over my life. I worked to constantly please others and be liked and accepted by them. I made it into the "in" crowd, but lost myself in the process. I also discovered that most of the "in" crowd "friends" weren't friends at all. Of course, how could they be? They didn't know the real me. It's taken time to regain a sense of who I am, but it all started with my faith and making a choice to be me. I had to stop hiding who I really was—and was meant to be—and break out of the façade I had been carrying around for so long. My arms and back were tired! Sometimes this means losing people you thought were your friends. Remember our healthy-living saboteurs?

When you can accept yourself for who you really are, right now—body, mind, and spirit—but also accept that there is room for improvement, you've taken a huge step in your journey towards wellness. You're on your way!

Stepping Stones

- Surrendering to your size means you have accepted the size you currently inhabit, and that is all.
- Size acceptance involves owning up to and accepting your current size, but moving forward from there to uncover your true size.
- Your true size is the size you are naturally meant to be—the size your body is happy being at, without having to do any unnatural or excessive things.
- Body acceptance is about taking the image we see and accepting it for what it is—being real about it.
- Nurture the areas of your body that drive you nuts!
- Celebrate your body as a whole and what it can do rather than just what it looks like.
- Accept your body, mind, and spirit as gifts.
- Your body, mind, and spirit are "on loan." Take care of them as well as you would anything you would borrow.
- Strive for a state of well-being, rather than a certain size or number on the scale.

PART TWO

Making Room
for Change

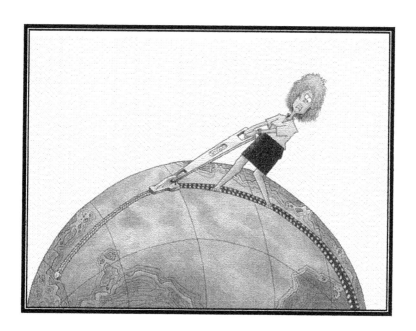

CHAPTER SIX

Self-Care, Self-Nurturing... or Self-Indulgence?

As women, we are nurturers. We see, hear, or smell a baby and that old nurturing instinct kicks in. Unfortunately, we often don't see the need to nurture ourselves. Why is that? There are several reasons, depending on our upbringing and circumstances. One of them may be because we've been taught that it's better to give than to receive (which I totally believe!). But wouldn't it be better to be able to give more, in more meaningful ways? Wouldn't it be great to be able to give abundantly? How do we do that? I believe that it's by taking care of ourselves.

Women are caregivers. We take care of everyone. And by the time we've taken care of everyone, we're just too darn tired to get out of our own way, let alone take care of ourselves. The kids get a bath, but we can't drag ourselves into the shower. We make sure their little faces are scrubbed glistening clean and hair is gelled and spiked or curled and ribboned, but we can't throw a little mascara and blush on our own faces, let alone get a comb through our hair. The kids each get their own plate at mealtime, but we just sort of pick off their leftovers or eat out of the pots and pans, wooden spoon and all (partly because it's one less dish

> "And that pretty much sums it up: we give ourselves the leftovers of life."

that needs to be washed!). And that pretty much sums it up: we give ourselves the leftovers of life.

But how can we give abundantly, when we're surviving on leftovers—and ones filled with artificial colors and preservatives, at that? We can't! Now, I'm not a believer in the "You've got to come first" or "You are your first priority" mantras. I see some men and women living by that little piece of advice, and they don't seem any happier than those of us living on leftovers. Neither end has any balance to it. Those living on leftovers are slowly draining their batteries. Those living by the "me-ism" philosophy do whatever they want, whenever they want, because, after all, if they're not happy, no one else will be either—and they'll make sure of that!

Living a life of balance, moderation, and wellness means taking care of yourself so that you can do what you have to do as well as you can do it. It means giving your body and spirit what they need, so you can then give to others in more meaningful, abundant ways. It means stepping back and taking a look at the molds you've been squeezing yourself into— molds that have been preventing you from being the best you...and in some cases, have prevented you from simply being yourself.

A Coaching Moment

Have you been living life on leftovers? What small gift of self-nurturing can you give yourself today?

I recently discovered my nails. Oh, I knew they were there, but being a writer, I don't need them. When they get too long, they just get in the way of my typing, interfering with my speed and agility at the keyboard.

They get in the way when I workout, too (try holding a dumbbell with daggers on the end of your fingers!). In general, I feel that having nails longer than the ends of my fingers are just a nuisance and get in the way. Normally, I would just clip them off (okay, okay, occasionally I bite them…but only when I'm desperate), or file them down, and away I'd go. Then there were the cuticles. Seems I always have at least one causing problems. When I was in college, I even had one become infected (right during finals—I even had to postpone an athletic training practical final, because I couldn't use my fingers to wrap and tape ankles. Talk about embarrassing!).

Not so long ago, one of my friends commented to another friend how beautiful her nails were. They weren't long…just, neat looking. Each little nail was the same length as the one next to it, and just looked, well, nice. I've never been into nail polish, and knew that wasn't for me, but as I discretely hid my own un-manicured digits from their view, I made a decision to rethink this whole nail thing. Should I be taking better care of them?

Before I could make the commitment to better nail health, I had to stop and think about whether I was making this leap out of pressure to fit into some mold—or did I just truly feel like I should be taking better care of my nails? I decided it was the latter. My cuticles were really ragged-looking and the hangnails…well, suffice it to say that they weren't a pretty site. But appearances aside, they often hurt and I didn't want to go through another bout of having one of them getting infected. So I've begun a small, simple ritual. It doesn't take a lot of time—or money. I bought some cuticle cream, and make more of a point to file my nails to about the same length and I push my cuticles back. It's far from being a manicure, and I would consider this more along the lines of simple self-care, but they look neater and healthier.

This brings me to a question. What is the difference between self-care and self-nurturing? And when does self-nurturing border on self-indulgence? And is self-indulgence a bad thing? Okay. That was three questions! But let's explore...

Self-Care... or Self-Nurturing?

One area I have always been very zealous with is shaving. My legs and armpits are shaved clean almost every night. I guess my biggest motivation to do this (other than not wanting to be mistaken for a contestant on "Survivor") is the thought that if I were ever in an accident, I wouldn't want the emergency crew to uncover a forest when they have to cut my clothes off. So imagine my surprise when I found out that not every woman feels this way! For myself, this is just a part of my normal self-care routine. But for other women, this is considered an indulgence—something they only do occasionally.

What activities are considered self-care? In my opinion, it's anything that would be considered normal, daily hygiene and grooming: brushing, flossing, bathing, hair care, skin care, cleaning ears... There are also weekly, monthly, and yearly self-care activities, too. Your monthly breast exam is an example of a monthly self-care event. Your annual pap is a yearly example.

But it's not quite that cut and dry. What one woman considers self-care, another would consider more of an indulgence. In my shaving example, I said that I consider shaving a part of my normal self-care routine—but other women wouldn't think so. I place working out under self-care, but for other women it's self-nurturing (or for some, self-torture!). Ironically, as I was working on this chapter, Oprah had a show about makeovers. Iman (one of the exotic super models) was one of the makeover givers, and they had a little blurb about her. For her, her weekly massage and facial is part of her self-care routine. She doesn't really consider it pampering, like many of us would (of course, when you own a multi-million dollar company, you can afford such luxuries!).

You see, there's a big gray area here. While I believe there are basic self-care activities, there are others that fall under either self-care or self-nurturing, depending on the person. What do I consider self-nurturing? For me, it's soaking in a hot bubble bath, lights dimmed, soft music playing, aromatherapy candles creating a soft glow. Or curling up with a good book by our fire, cup of tea nearby. And while I consider working out a part of my normal self-care routine, I realize that it also has many self-nurturing properties. Talk about a gray area!

So, is self-nurturing necessary (I guess that adds another question to our list!)? Absolutely. (We'll discuss in a moment why I think so.) I also believe that self-care and self-nurturing are inter-locked. Picture two conjoining rings. While each one is its own ring, they also can't be separated. Self-care routines have self-nurturing properties, and many self-nurturing activities should be a part of your self-care routine. At the other end of the spectrum, many self-indulgent activities can also have self-nurturing properties. While I would consider a weekly facial indulgent (due in part to our financial status), I realize that it would also have self-nurturing properties. It would give me some time to myself, be relaxing, and help me feel good about taking care of my skin. In this case, is it wrong to indulge? That depends on a few things…which we'll get to in a minute. But I think we answered our second question: when does self-nurturing border on self-indulgence.

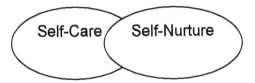

A Coaching Moment

What do you consider to be your basic, grooming, self-care needs? Make a list of them, including things you don't currently do, but think should be done. Separate them into daily, weekly, monthly, and yearly activities. How many of these necessities are you keeping up on? Choose one or two you'd like to start incorporating into your routine on a regular basis. Set up your goals, make an action plan, and begin today to start meeting your basic needs.

Should we feel guilty for doing what many of us would consider normal grooming or self-care? We claim to not have the time for simple grooming, like filing our nails or applying a little make-up. We don't shave until we have to. Our hair goes up into a ponytail every day, because we don't have time to do anything with it. We don't have time to properly brush and floss, but then end up spending hours in the dentist's chair. See where I'm going here? As women, we must at least take care of our basic, minimal needs, so that we can be more giving in more meaningful ways.

84

Now let's explore how you view things on your self-nurturing list, like bubble baths, curling up with a good book and a cup of tea, or having lunch with a friend. Let's pretend for a moment, that time isn't a factor here. Would you still take the time to do these types of activities for yourself? Or would there be too much guilt attached?

I'm the first to admit that as women and mothers, we are in a tough position. We're supposed to go on date nights with our husbands on a regular basis. We're supposed to give our kids quality and quantity time. We may have clients or family or neighbors or friends all vying for our time and attention—not to mention our poor neglected homes. If you're single, you may feel more obliged to be the co-worker who works late, takes on extra projects, goes on the business trips, and volunteers for the board meetings, because you don't have children or a spouse who require your attention. And this is where the whole de-cluttering theme comes in—getting rid of the "fluff." It's really very difficult to move forward in the self-nurturing process until we've done some house and schedule cleaning. By freeing up some time, it's easier to allow ourselves to be nurtured—without the guilt attached.

A Coaching Moment

What do you need to do to give yourself some nurturing time? How do you feel about the thought of giving yourself this gift? Do you feel you're worth it? Take some time to journal your thoughts. Write down some activities you would find self-nurturing. Choose one. How could you incorporate this one thing into your life sometime in the next month?

Begin to make a plan and stick with it. And choose not to feel guilty for it.

So, is indulging in activities a bad thing? I admit that I've had to do some thinking on this subject myself. Some believe that any indulgence is bad, and is really based on self-hate. The definition here of indulgence would be partaking in a harmful activity, such as binging on your local supermarket's flavor-of-the-month—which just happens to be your favorite flavor. Personally, I see this more as *over*indulgence. But let's look at this rationally. Webster defines indulgence as "to give free rein to, to take unrestrained pleasure in." That's the first definition. The second definition is, "to yield to the desire of, to treat with excessive leniency, generosity, or consideration." One of the synonyms Webster uses is "to pamper."

Starting with the first definition, one would think that maybe indulging isn't such a great idea. I mean, "unrestrained pleasure" sounds sort of, well, like it could really get you into trouble! And that's the definition that things like binging or getting a little carried away at your best friend's bachelorette party would fall under. These things aren't healthy, and they aren't based on self-love or taking care of yourself.

Going by the second definition, it sort of softens things a bit. The confusing thing is that we use words like "indulge," "pamper," and "self-nurture" interchangeably. It's not till you allow Mr. Webster to officially define the terms that we realize that maybe we've been using the terms incorrectly.

At first glance, the second definition doesn't seem bad at all—until you focus on the word "excessive." Excessive anything isn't a good thing, even for things that are supposed to be good for you. Too much water can be deadly, after all. But

honestly, used the way we use these terms today, I don't see
the harm in occasionally doing something you normally
wouldn't do—like book a professional massage—as long as
you don't have to sell your firstborn in order to afford it, or
totally "dis" your husband in the process. And it should be a
healthy "indulgence." I also feel it's healthy to, say, order
dessert while you're eating out at your favorite restaurant. Or
treat yourself to seasonal goodies during the holidays—as long
as you use balance and moderation. To try to deny yourself this
pleasure will most likely lead to overindulgence.

So I don't see the word indulgence as a bad thing, as long
as it is used with moderation, balance, common sense, and a
sense of well-being. Maybe we should re-word it…how about
healthy indulgences? Or healthy pampering? What about
luxury? That's a good one. Webster defines luxury as,
"something adding to pleasure or comfort but not absolutely
necessary." That really defines what we're taking about here.
On the other hand, the very next definition says, "an
indulgence in something that provides pleasure, satisfaction, or
ease." So there you go! We can't seem to get away from it, can
we?

A Coaching Moment

What activities do you consider to be indulgences or
luxuries? Think about why you feel that way. List the reasons
why you wouldn't occasionally participate in such activities.
Which activities that you've listed are healthy and would
contribute to your well-being? Is the reason you gave for not
doing it good enough? If the reason has more to do with
guilt and feeling undeserving, journal your thoughts.

Bringing the Spa Home

A visit to the spa can do wonders to lift your spirits. But when you walk out the door, you leave the spa behind. Solution? Bring the spa home!

Okay, I know what you're thinking—I can't afford that! But I'm not talking about remodeling your bathroom into your own private spa. No, I'm talking about some very simple, inexpensive ways to give yourself royal treatment that won't break the bank.

Create a Sanctuary: First things first—pick a spot in your home and make it your own. Try to choose a spot that is out of the flow of traffic and will be as free of distractions and clutter as possible. "You should have a place you can retreat to," says Paula McClure, owner of the Mood Spa in Dallas, Texas. "It can be as simple as a comfortable chair surrounded by some of your favorite things—like pictures or a good cup of herbal tea. This should be a place for you to meditate, pray, or write your favorite thoughts in your journal."

Set the Mood: Our moods can take us on a rollercoaster ride; all the more reason to create a mood that is soft and relaxing. There are several ways to do this, depending upon the type of experience you're looking for.

The Mood of Fragrance: Scents have a unique effect on the body. Some are cool and calming; others are zippy and stimulating. Scents are not universal in their acceptance, however, as what one person will think is delish, another will find downright irritating.

"One of the joys, as well as one of the frustrations," says Donna Maria, aromatherapist and author *of Making Aromatherapy Creams and Lotions* (Storey Books, 2000), "is that aromatherapy is different for everyone. It's very subjective."

The Mood of Music: We all know that music can set a mood. Research has even shown that music affects the brain's pleasure centers that govern moods and emotions. Throw on some Michael Jackson and you'll be up on your feet boogying. Slide in Michael Bolton, though, and you're set for an evening of romance. What kind of music is considered relaxing is also subjective. Perhaps it's classical that does it for you, or maybe a symphony of nature sounds. To try some very soothing spa music, check out what Champion Press has available at www.championpress.com Click on GIFT IDEAS and take a look at the SPA CD Set or the Enlightenment set.

The Mood of Lighting: When we want to relax, we don't sit under glaring-bright lights. So dim the lamps and light a few candles—make them aromatherapy candles and you take care of two steps!

Choose Your Ammunition: Okay, you've got your space and you've set the mood. Now what? This will vary depending on what your needs are at the time. Here are some possibilities:

Do nothing! When was the last time someone told you to do that?! Actually, doing nothing is really doing a lot. While relaxed and calm, your body releases some pretty powerful hormones. These endorphins block pain receptors, that in turn decrease your sense of pain. They also give you an overall feeling of well-being.

Hit the tub. Soaking in a nice warm tub can do wonders for you. Add a few drops of an essential oil or bubble bath.

Slather yourself in sheer luxury. To slough off that dead dry skin, Olga Morales from the Red Door Spa, recommends mixing sea salts with oil and gently rubbing the mixture all over your body. Rinse and follow with a sheer, light lotion, or a thick, rich cream—your call.

Do some journaling. Remember that little sanctuary? Now is the perfect time to snuggle in and write down your thoughts and feelings. Research shows that doing this acts as a stress-reliever.

Massahhhhhhge. Massage can be a great relaxant, although some women will find that they tense up during it depending on their "masseuse" (men can get a little carried away sometimes!). If this is the case, speak up and ask your masseuse to ease up a bit. Remember, effleurage means light, feather-like strokes. Say it—"efffffluerrrrragggge." Sounds light, doesn't it?

No matter what your schedule, pencil in some time that is all yours. It can be as little as five minutes if that's all you've got (see next page for Paula McClure's suggestions). And don't forget to nurture the inside of yourself, too. Eating healthy, wholesome foods and keeping hydrated with plenty of pure fluids is really the first step in self-nurturing.

And if you absolutely, positively feel that you have no time for any sort of pampering routine, you could do what Michelle Smith started while she was pregnant: her "daily little-bit-of-chocolate rule." Mmmmm. We're all familiar with chocolate's pampering effects—not to mention that current research shows that cocoa contains disease-fighting antioxidants. But we didn't need research to prove this to us—we women knew it was healthy all along!

No Time?

Paula McClure recommends creating a mini-retreat and giving yourself a pampering quickie when you're short on time!

5 Minute
Try a self-massage. Sit cross-legged and warm a small amount of oil in your hands—vegetable, olive, sesame, or almond oils are all great. A drop or two of essential oil makes a wonderful addition. Massage your neck, shoulders, and hands with circular, then small tapping movements. Your face can also be done at this time.

10 Minute
Relax with a foot soak and scrub. Fill a bucket with warm water and add a few drops of your favorite shower gel. Soak for about five minutes. Remove one foot and scrub with either a commercial exfoliant, or make your own with sea salt and oil. After doing both feet, rinse, pat dry, and apply a moisturizer.

15 Minute
Give yourself a steamy rose petal facial. Start with a clean face. Place fresh rose petals in a large bowl and pour nearly boiling water over them. Add three drops of lavender oil. Lean over the steam with a towel draped over your head, approximately 9-12 inches away for 10 minutes to open up pores, moisturize skin, and stimulate circulation. Follow-up with a mask or exfoliant and moisturizer.

Stepping Stones

- It's imperative to balance-out living life on leftovers and living by a me-ism philosophy.
- Self-care is grooming and hygiene.
- While self-care and self-nurturing are each distinctive, they also overlap.
- Self-nurturing is not an optional part of living a life of wellness.
- Some of the things we call indulgences are really just simple self-nurturing.

CHAPTER SEVEN

All Stressed Out
And Nowhere to Go

One area most of us tend to ignore is stress. But it's
also one that if you're to get started on your journey,
is a necessary thing to face—and take care of.

Stress is a funny thing. When asked if we're stressed out,
many of us could answer that our lives define the word stress.
Just look "stress" up in the dictionary and there we are! Others
will claim they have no stress...but they have their token two
drinks a night (it's relaxing), have stomach problems (just a
little irritable bowel), and then there's this little eye-twitching
annoyance (but it's only a problem while driving).

Chances are, we all have stress in our lives. And not all
stress is bad. A little stress keeps us invigorated, alive. At
times, stress can be a motivator. But when it becomes
overwhelming, it can have some pretty serious consequences.
Experts now tell us that stress can be the root of many a
disease, including cancer, heart disease, asthma, and
gastrointestinal problems. It can also contribute to depression,
anger problems, and loss of short-term memory.

Okay, that last one is sort of my own interpretation based
on experience. But think about it. We rush around, going from
one event to the next, barely having time to pee, let alone eat.
There's no time to focus on one thing. How many times have
we gone to the store to get a specific item, only to realize when
we get home that we totally forgot to get the one thing we went

to the store for in the first place? And how many of us have
forgotten a child at practice or rehearsal? They suddenly show
up on the doorstep, after having one of the "really organized,
stress-free moms" notice that their ride hadn't arrived and offer
to bring them home ("That poor thing."). If this hasn't
happened to you yet, just wait. It will! It all starts at the
moment of conception, when those little brain suckers begin
sapping brain cells from you—brain cells that are gone forever!
Then after they're born, it just continues to go downhill, as
you're now responsible for someone other than yourself. I
mean, it's difficult enough just having to get yourself ready.
And if you breastfeed – forget it! Did you know there's a
direct connection from your brain to your breasts? Really!
Anyway, where was I? Oh yeah. Stress…

How is Your Stress Packaged?

Stress can come in many different packages. There's the kind
of stress that would make any of us frazzled, what I like to call
"universal stress"—things like natural disasters, for instance.
There aren't too many of us that wouldn't freak out if a tornado
was heading in our direction. Death of a loved one is another
one. Even if the death was on some level a relief (due to some
conflict in the relationship or because the loved one was
suffering greatly), there is still great stress involved—whether
or not we show much emotion at the time. The thing with stress
is that it can be shoved deep down inside of us. Oh yeah. We
look like we're handling life just hunky dory on the outside.
People comment on how amazed they are that we're managing
life as well as we are given the circumstances. But we know.
We know what secrets we're hiding deep down in our guts. We
fight to keep them there, because they're just ready to burst, but

we continue to wrestle them down anyway. And what happens? We find that we're always getting sick. We readily get colds, flu bugs, cooties—or something much more serious, in the form of chronic illness. You see, the stress seeps out one way or another. Whether we choose to ignore it or stuff it, it will find a way out.

A Coaching Moment

Are you often sick? Do you suffer from a chronic illness? Do a stress inventory and pinpoint your major sources of stress.

Stress is also based on our perception of things. It's the old "one man's trash is another man's treasure" phenomenon. What one person considers very stressful, another one thinks is no big deal. As an example, you've taken your kids (or your nieces and nephews or your friend's kids…) out for lunch to a restaurant (something other than a fast food store), and, although they've behaved very well, they accidentally spill their drink—all over them, all over you, all over the couple sitting next to you. How do you react? I see two choices here. The person who perceives this as a normal event with children will apologize to the couple, start sopping up the mess with any available napkins, call the waiter over for more napkins (or a mop), and order another drink—with a cover this time. The person who sees this as, "Oh my gosh! I can't believe this happened! I'm so embarrassed! Why did I bring you here? I told you to be careful with that cup! I'm so, soooo sorry… " is probably on the verge of a nervous breakdown, and will not have any remaining enjoyable time while at the restaurant. Part of this is because they're too busy worrying about what everyone is thinking about them. Did you notice how many times the word "I" was used in the above scenario? Hmmmm. As we discussed previously, it ends up boiling down to a choice. You can change your perception of what you consider stressful by simply choosing to do so. Of course, there is some conditioning that must be done. It will take some practice—and constant reminding that this is what you're choosing. After all, whether it's a cognitive change or a behavioral one, there is a learning curve involved. Learning and applying stress-management techniques can also help ease you into this new mindset. More on that in a minute.

Another root of our stress is homes and schedules. They can literally make us sick. The other day I was speaking with a friend, and she sounded down. When I asked her what was wrong, she said that she just felt overwhelmed, and needed to spend some time that weekend de-cluttering her closets. That was part of her solution to feeling better—and a good one at that.

Look around you. Does your home give you a good feeling? Or does it send icy chills up your spine and make you want to bulldoze the whole house down so you don't have to look at it anymore? Even if you have "clean clutter" and "know right where everything is," does it embarrass you to have others over, because they may not understand and think you're a total slob? Does it still stress you out just having all this stuff to contend with? And what about your schedule? Does it allow time for you to do anything you enjoy? Or is it filled with

> Do you feel like you're constantly on a time clock, determining the minutes you have before the next event? Do you have time to cook nutritious meals? Or is hitting a different drive-through each night your idea of eating a variety of foods?

work, meetings, running here and there? Do you feel like you're constantly on a time clock, determining the minutes you have before the next event? Do you have time to cook nutritious meals? Or is hitting a different drive-through each night your idea of eating a variety of foods? Do you have any down time at all, or are you constantly on the go all day long, and the only break you get is when your head hits the pillow? And that's only assuming everyone stays in their beds that night.

Ladies! Something has got to give! The stress in our lives is making us sick—physically, mentally, emotionally, and spiritually. When we are too busy to cook a meal for our neighbor who just had a baby or offer to take a co-worker's kids for a few hours so she can spend time with her ill father who's in the hospital, we're too busy. When we become so busy that we don't have time for others, let alone ourselves, we lose out on one of the things that makes us human—the relational aspect of life. When we don't have time to take care of ourselves, how can we possibly expect to have enough to give to others?

One of the huge, overlying causes of stress is trying to squeeze ourselves into molds that don't fit. These molds can come in many shapes and sizes.

One mold that comes to mind is whether or not to work after having children. Maybe your spouse or your in-laws or your own parents or your friends expect you to work. And so you do. You return back to work fulltime, after three wonderful, fulfilling months at home with your new baby. Even you are surprised at how much you enjoyed being at home. And while you like your job and also find it fulfilling, the added stress is killing you. You're constantly exhausted.

You have no time to do any of the things you enjoy, such as cooking or pleasure reading. Workout? Fuhgedaboudit! And while your husband expects you to work, he's not expected to help out any more around the house. Have I just described you? Pretty close?

The first thing you must realize, when it comes to trying to break out of a mold, is that you do have options! I know. Been there, done that. Is it easy? No! Is it worth it? Yes! You must get out of the all-or-nothing frame of mind. So many mothers think they have to work fulltime or not at all. And since the budget demands you must work, you work. But there are other options: part-time work, job sharing, working from home, working a different shift or cutting back family expenses. This can also work, by the way, with fulltime stay-at-home moms. You're expected to stay at home, and so you do. However, you can't help but think that just a day or two out of the house would do you some good, which in turn would be reflected in the job you're doing at home. And so the tug-of-war ensues.

You must find your own personal and family balance, regardless of what others' expectations are of you. Of course, whole books have been written on the working mom/stay-at-home mom thing. I don't intend to cause a stir with this book about these issues. I do, however, hope to get to you to think about this issue, because it is such a huge part of a woman's life. Is your current personal situation beneficial to you? Is it beneficial to your children? Do you need to make some changes? Or is it time for you to finally make peace with what you're doing?

A Coaching Moment

In what ways are you feeling squeezed into someone else's mold? What would be some other options to what you're currently doing?

I had this struggle when I first decided to stay at home. I guess, growing up in my generation, that I always assumed I'd have to work. My mom didn't work while we were young, though, so I had the advantage of having the role model to stay at home. But my first few years were rough. I knew I wanted to be home—but part of me still longed for the outside stimulation I had gotten from work. I didn't want the hassle of daycare and missing out on the intimacy I could have with my children. I had returned to work after my first son was born, and although I had a near-perfect set-up (I cut my hours to 30 a week, my husband's aunt watched my son, and I was able to leave to nurse him on my lunch break), there were still things about the baby that she knew and I didn't—like what time his naps were. And this bothered me. So after our second son was born, I stayed home. But for years, I allowed the tug-of-war to steal my joy of being at home during their early years. It wasn't until I made peace with it all—embraced where I was at the time—that I was able to relax and be at peace with where I was —at home.

Let's take a look now to see what's really stressing you out, and what you need to do to make peace.

How Do You Spell S-t-r-e-s-s?

Most of us never slow down long enough to think about what it is that's really stressing us out. We just know that we're

STRESSED OUT! It's important to uncover what your main stressors are and how you react to them in order to change your behavior. So stop for a moment. Think about what really stresses you out.

Stress-Savers

1. Identify your stressors.
2. Pinpoint what exactly about them is the problem.
3. Can they be controlled?
   If yes, what do you need to do to manage them?
   Take action? Change your reaction?
4. Change your perception of those stressors that can't be changed themselves. Consider making peace with your situation, especially if it's an on-going, long-lasting one. Ask yourself if there is anything that can be done the next time to avoid getting into the current situation.
5. Learn to deal with those stressors that are just stressful to you, period, by using coping mechanisms.

A Coaching Moment

Make a list of your major stressors, as well as your corresponding reactions to them. Break each stressor down. What aspect of each one is really the problem? For instance, if one of your stressors is your job, what exactly about it is stressful? Is it the hours? Your co-workers? The location? Your boss? The whole job? Pinpoint what really is the problem within the general stressor, then decide if it's something you can control. This can be tricky, because at first glance, you may think there's nothing you can do about it. But chances are, there are several steps you can take, or at least attempt. In this case, can you change your hours? Can you work part-time? Does this company have other locations that would be closer to your home? Do you need to confront a co-worker? Do you need to consider changing jobs? Brainstorm reasonable, realistic solutions to your source of stress. Then make a plan to take action.

Sometimes stressors can be a bit more gray in nature. Let's take in-laws, for instance. If you have in-law woes, you may think there isn't a whole lot you can do about it (short of ending up on America's Most Wanted!). But brainstorm a while.

> Have you ever noticed that the word "desserts" is "stressed" spelled backwards? Or is it the other way around?

What about the relationship can be changed? Concentrate on what you can change, since as we know, we can't change anyone other than ourselves. Again, pinpoint what the problem is. Let's say they tend to be overbearing and try to take-over (do I see anyone nodding her head?). Okay. So you know how they are. Now think about how you react to them. Do you become defensive? Do you just clam up, since it isn't worth saying anything anyway? Be honest about your reaction. Now brainstorm different, healthier reactions. If you tend to become defensive, would it hurt to just keep your mouth shut sometimes, especially if what you say doesn't make a difference anyway or always comes out the wrong way? If you tend to clam up, are there times when you should speak up and be more assertive? This is important when what they're doing or saying affects your children or your relationship with your husband. Many times, you need to start with yourself and your own reaction when your stress involves other people.

What about those stressors that can't be controlled at all? What then? You have a choice to change your perception of the

101

situation. This is where how one views certain events determines the reaction to it. If you don't view the situation as stressful to begin with, then there's no problem. For this example, let's use traffic. How does getting stuck in traffic affect your mood? Do you accept it as one of those nothing-I-can-do-about-it things, and consider it a good time to get caught up on all those forgotten Kegels (and you thought they were just for pregnancy!)? Or does your breathing immediately become shallow, your heart start racing, words you forbid your children to say come out of your mouth, fists pound the dash board, horn's 'a honkin'? Wouldn't it be better in situations where you have no control to just surrender and go with the flow? Even if it means you're going to be late to your appointment or will get home later? If you're going to be late no matter what your reaction, why not change your perception and relax?

There is another side to this story, too. Maybe you're not just reacting to the current situation. Maybe you're angry with yourself for not leaving earlier or taking a different route. You see, even in the midst of situations we can't control, there may be some aspect of control to the "big picture." Which all goes back to being more organized, planning ahead, and de-cluttering home and schedule. Are you beginning to see how this is all connected?

There may be some things in your life that just stress you out, period, no matter what you do about them. You've tried and tried to change how you react; you've tried to pretend they don't make you burn inside to the point you're wondering if smoke is literally pouring out your ears. What do you do then? You learn to deal or cope with these stressful situations.

Rate-a-Stress Level

If stress is really a nemesis to you, it's helpful to set goals related to stress-management techniques and actions, such as writing at least three journal entries a week. It's also useful to rate your stress level. This can be done using a simple 1-10 scale, 10 being "ready to have a nervous breakdown," and 1 being "constantly in a state of total serenity." First, choose a number-goal that you would like your stress-rating to average. Let's pick 3. Then, at the end of each day, rate your stress level for that day. At the end of the week, average your ratings. Did you come close to your goal?

Stress management has been a popular buzz-word among the health and fitness crowd for some time now. Stress-management coping techniques are wonderful tools to use for those times when we need to de-stress and have no other options. My only word of caution, though, is that they can sometimes be used as a bandage to a situation that really requires surgery. It's like a doctor who keeps prescribing medication, without ever looking into and treating the root of the problem. So I encourage you to first go through the steps on page 106—action, reaction, and perception—to deal with the roots, and use coping techniques when there are no other options. The following techniques can be used by themselves or in any combination.

Take a deep breath in...and out. Deep breathing is one of the most simple, most "portable" techniques available, since it can be done anywhere, anytime, and doesn't require a Ph.D. to understand. When we get stressed out, we tend to breath very shallowly, using just the top part of our lungs. Deep breathing helps to calm us, sending oxygen to the deepest part of our lungs, and therefore, increasing oxygen to the rest of our bodies.

The instructions are simple: breathe in deeply through your nose, and slowly exhale through your mouth. Some people find a relaxed mouth to work best, others prefer to sort of purse their lips to slow down the breath. Then again, if you're into yoga, you may know that the old yogis recommend breathing both in and out through your nose. Do what works for you.

Think...coooool. Imagining cool, calming colors can invite a peaceful, relaxing feeling to take over. Bright, fiery colors, such as red, orange, and yellow, tend to be more tense-producing hues, whereas cool colors—blue, green, purple—evoke a feeling of calm. Simply closing your eyes and picturing these colors in your head can bring the stress level down.

Imagine that! Visualizing cool colors is a form of mental imagery or visualization. But mental imagery can go way beyond just colors. By "placing" yourself in a peaceful, relaxing environment—what I like to call, your special place—you can calm yourself down. Your special place might be a warm, sandy beach, a favorite room or a mountain top—wherever you feel at most peace. Sometimes, going back to a favorite childhood spot may end up being your special place. Remember that tree house?

1, 2, buckle my shoe. Sometimes, all we need are a few seconds to cool down. Counting to ten can give you the time you need to cool the overheated jets and think more rationally. This comes in handy when one of your kids breaks your great-

great-great grandmother's antique tea set. Or, you're handed the bill to have your oil changed and you find out they took it upon themselves to also change the brakes, the spark plugs, and every fluid that flows through a vehicle's veins. Some people like counting down from ten. This is fine. Although for me personally, it feels more like a countdown to take-off, and makes me want to do just that—explode like a rocket ship.

Relax, relax! When we get stressed out, our muscles tense up. Progressive relaxation can be done when you need a quick stress check, or if you have more time, you can do a total relaxation. Get in a position where your muscles aren't supporting any part of your body—you can totally sink into the floor or whatever it is you're lying on. Part of progressive relaxation is sensing the difference between a tensed up muscle and a relaxed one. To do this, start by clenching your fists as tightly as you can; then totally relax them. Repeat this action— purposely tensing the muscles and then letting them go—do several muscle groups. Then, starting at the top of your head, slowly move down your body, being especially aware of your muscles, relaxing each one and allowing all the tension to flow outward. Take a deep breath every now and then, and visualize the stress and tension leaving your body as you exhale. You can also combine this with visualization of your special place. Total relaxation can last as long as you want it to. It's a great tool to use for those nights when you're having a tough time falling asleep, too. Or, if you've been short on sleep lately, experts say that 20 minutes of deep relaxation can equal two hours of sleep! Yee ha! Talk about multitasking!

Let's say, however, that you don't have the time to do a total relaxation, but you just need a quick stress check. Do the tense-relax sequence down your body so your muscles get a sense of the difference. Then take a moment to relax your entire body—if you're sitting in a chair, allow your upper body to fall forward to your lap and your arms to just hang—deep breathe, and even bring yourself to your special place. End by inhaling while bringing your arms overhead; slowly lower your arms while exhaling.

A Coaching Moment

Which one of the previous stress-coping mechanisms works best for you? How can you remind yourself to practice it the next time you get in a stressful situation?

Stress Management Maintenance Plan

In order to consistently manage your stress, it helps to include activities in your life that are calming to your spirit. These types of activities are as varied and subjective as stress is. While one activity may totally relax and invigorate one person, it might totally stress another out. So I'm going to give you some ideas to work with. Choose some that appeal to you, and add others that fit you personally. You may notice, that these options cover the whole you: mentally, emotionally, physically, and spiritually.

Work it out. Or maybe I should say, workout it out. Exercising, whether it's cardio, strength training, or stretching, for many people, is relaxing. Of course, there's yoga, which many find calms them and brings them down to a more peaceful state. But even something like kickboxing, where you can literally punch and kick out your frustrations on an imaginary opponent or punching bag, can be a great stress reliever. And hey, better that bag than your neighbor!

Journal it out. Writing your feelings and frustrations down on paper can be very cathartic. Think back to when you were a young girl. Did you have a diary? Wasn't it helpful to write out your feelings? Even journaling has made it into the research realm. One study found that people with rheumatoid arthritis who journaled had a lessening of their symptoms. Think about that. Journaling has both psychological and physical benefits! One great thing about journaling that I've found is that it encourages you to find solutions. It's one thing to just think it in your head. It's another to actually see your problems on paper, and write down possible solutions.

Pray it out. Praying and giving your problems and needs over to One who is greater than any of us can be very freeing. It's that whole surrendering thing. Recognizing that God is ultimately in control, and that there are times when all we have is Him, is a necessary ingredient to living in wellness. When you come up against roadblocks in your path, why not try asking Him for direction? Better yet, why not ask Him throughout the entire journey? When worry and anxiety are overtaking your spirit, make a choice to give them to Him. Worrying will not gain anything—except maybe a big ol' migraine. Surrender to the One who knows you better than anyone else, and who can give you all that you need.

Ahhhh it out. When was the last time you had a bubble bath? Have you ever had a professional massage? What about a facial? A trip to the local day spa? Most of us don't take the time to pamper ourselves. And in fact, many of us would say to take that time would cause more stress, as we'd feel guilty for taking time for ourselves—especially on something so unnecessary. There is also the obstacle of guilt when we spend money on "extras" for ourselves. It all comes back, though, to taking care of ourselves so we have more to give to others. If money is tight, I'm not suggesting you go and spend your entire savings on yourself. There are little nurturing things you can do that cost just pennies—a bubble bath, for instance, or a facial mask.

A Coaching Moment
How can you begin incorporating a lifelong stress-management plan? What is your first step in doing so?

Stepping Stones
- Stress can affect every part of you.
- How you deal with your stress will depend on what kind of stress it is and its source.
- Identify the source of your stress.
- Pinpoint what it is about the general source that stresses you out.
- Determine if it's something that can be controlled— then act.
- If it can't be controlled, try changing either your reaction to, or perception of it.
- Consider making peace with where you're at and embracing where you're at in your life.
- For those stressors where nothing can be changed, learn and apply some of the stress management techniques within this chapter.

CHAPTER EIGHT
Mission: Dumping the Clutter Bug

You may be wondering why I have a chapter on de-cluttering in a book about wellness. First of all, clutter, whether it's a cluttered schedule (what I call a "fluffy" schedule) or a cluttered home, is all baggage that needs to be dumped in order to really begin your journey. Plus, it's just so practical. How many times have you read, "You just need to make the time to workout," and you're thinking, "When?!" I mean,

> I like the notion that a de-cluttered home plus a de-cluttered schedule will bring you a more de-cluttered spirit.

c'mon! Every night of the week is taken up with something—some meeting, a ball game, a recital, practice, rehearsal...and if there is a night or weekend where there's nothing, it's catch-up time, trying to take care of everything else that doesn't get done the rest of the time! This chapter is meant to help with the time excuse.

I like the notion that "a de-cluttered home plus a de-cluttered schedule will bring you a more de-cluttered spirit." By weeding out those things in our lives that do not add to our growth, it allows us more opportunities to concentrate on those things that do. Therefore, I'm also including it to, hopefully, help you exterminate the phrase, "I don't have enough time to workout (to cook healthy homemade meals, to take a bubble bath—whatever!)" from your vocabulary.

If there's one thing in life that we're all on a level playing field with, it's time. Although some of us would like to believe we must have fewer hours than everyone else, in reality we each have a full 24 hours each day—no more, no less. It's what you do with that time that makes the difference. So since we're on the subject, let's begin by delving into this issue and doing a little schedule-de-cluttering. Shall we?

Just Say No!

This little phrase became a part of our culture when former First Lady, Nancy Reagan, dubbed it the slogan for the drug war campaign. Some of us may remember it from having our parents pound it into our brains. Or, depending on your age, you were the one doing the pounding. But this phrase isn't appropriate for just drugs. It can be applied to many other areas of our lives as well.

We've already discussed somewhat, how most of us fill our lives with so much "stuff." (Remember the "fluff" at the expense of more meaningful things?) We justify material "stuff" by saying that we need it, it serves a purpose—or at least will serve a purpose some day when we might need it (or have time to use it). Then we cram our schedules so full of "stuff" that we barely have time to use the bathroom. A best friend just had a baby and it would be nice to take over a meal or offer to take her older kids for a while, but who's got the time? Time to cook decent, healthy meals? As long as it comes from a box! Exercise? Does walking upstairs to bed at night count? Ah, but we've got good reason for this, too. All that time we spend volunteering for those fifteen different committees and organizations just proves how giving and helpful we are. And after all, if we don't do it, who will?

Ladies! It's time to hang up your capes and retire your Super Woman suits. It's time to start enjoying your home, your families—your life! It's time to be joyful! And it's time to start saying no. Saying no is tough, but it's a necessity if you're to live a life of wellness.

A Coaching Moment

In what ways do you try to have it all? Do you believe a woman can truly have it all, all at once? Or does it come in various seasons? Can a woman have it all and do it all well? Journal your thoughts.

As an example, a friend and I were talking recently. Her son was playing basketball (among other activities), and our boys were not. She wanted to know how we did it.

"How do you do it? How do you say no?" she asked.

"Simple," I replied. "I open my mouth..." Okay, so it's not really that simple. Remember earlier when we discussed our journey on a motor home? What was the first thing we needed? Desire. Right? In this case, we didn't want to confine our entire winter— weekends and all—to basketball and driving, sometimes for two hours, in winter weather.

Next, you need to make a choice—either go with what you desire, or choose what you know in the end will not make you happy. We chose to not do basketball. As it is, our boys do soccer, skiing, and baseball for sports, and we thought that was plenty. We didn't see any benefit to adding basketball to the schedule.

The next step is to make a plan. In our situation, we planned an alternative activity. Since we live in the Northeast, they do outdoor activities in the winter instead—and don't suffer because of missing out on basketball. We also had to plan to stick with our decision!

Finally, you need to act on your decision. That's where actually saying "no" comes in. If you live in a small town, you understand the pressure for your kids to be involved in everything. And because everyone knows everyone, small town people really have a knack for slathering on the guilt when you decline. But you need to decide what is best for you and your family, not what's in the town's best interest. You'll need to come to a point in your life where you feel good rather than guilty for saying no. Obviously, there are times we have to say no to something we really wish we could say yes to. But so much of our lives is filled with fulfilling other people's expectations of us (the "mold"). In our case, saying no definitely paid off. The parents whose kids played basketball complained all season long because of the crazy schedule. Weeknights and every weekend were eaten up with basketball. Some games were more than two hours away. And some days, they had a game in the morning and another game somewhere else in the afternoon. Did I mention these were nine-year-olds?

Learning to say no is one of the first steps in living a life in wellness and building the healthy life you and your family deserve. Yes, there are things that we have to do that don't necessarily instill a warm fuzzy feeling (can't say as I love the mounds of daily laundry and dishes!), although we can choose to change our attitudes about those things, too. The "extras" that you choose to fill your life with—do they bring you joy? Or do you dread that weekly meeting? Do you absolutely hate your job? Or do you flit out of the house each morning, merrily anticipating another day at the office? Okay, maybe that's a little much, but you get the idea. Having a bunch of junk crammed into our lives that we loathe can also color other things. For instance, maybe it's not really exercise that you hate. Maybe you think you hate it because you don't have the time to workout the way you need to, to enjoy it. So instead, you resort to the dreaded stationary bike because it's right there and available and put in your time—as little of it as possible!

Some of you may have to actually practice saying no. Try role-playing with a friend or your spouse. Come up with various situations that you have encountered in the past or that you know you will encounter in the future. Have your partner pretend to be the person trying to get you to join a committee or make costumes for the next school play or take on a more time-consuming position in an organization you already belong to. Come up with a few different ways you can gently—and honestly—turn the offer down.

> Having a bunch of junk crammed into our lives that we loathe can also color other things. For instance, maybe it's not really exercise that you hate. Maybe you think you hate it because you don't have the time to workout the way you need to, to enjoy it.

Once you've done this, you now have some ammunition in your back pocket that you can pull out when offered or asked to do something you feel you can't.

A Coaching Moment

In what areas of your life do you need to practice saying "No" to?

Living Life On Purpose— Not By Accident

Tell me—what's your purpose in life? Why were you put on this planet? Don't know? Most of us don't ever really consider this question. Hey—life happens! Right? Our tendency is to get so caught up in life, with no real direction. We may know we want a bigger house, a nicer car, a new wardrobe…and so we base what we do on what we want. But does this fulfill your purpose in life?

Everyone has a purpose, a reason, for being. You weren't a mistake, accidentally dropped off here by some stork. You have a reason for being here. If you know your purpose, then you have no excuse for not living life on purpose—and therefore, I'm afraid to tell you, the whole time issue shouldn't be an issue. If you're living life according to your purpose in life, then your life will be filled with the things that fulfill that requirement. You will choose to fill your life with those things that fulfill your purpose. Make sense? You won't have a schedule filled with "fluff," because everything you do will matter to you.

If, on the other hand, you don't know your purpose in life, I encourage you to find it! There are some great books on this topic, which I list in the "Good Reads" section of this book, but a couple I'd like to mention now are *Passion on Purpose: Discovering and Pursuing a Life that Matters* by Dr. Deborah Newman and *The Purpose Driven Life: What on Earth am I Here For?* by Rick Warren. The first one is written specifically for women, and is a great place to start that leg of your journey.

A Coaching Moment

What's your purpose in life? What are your gifts, talents, and interests? Usually, your purpose will overlap these things.

> One other thing I encourage you to do is consider each of your children's true gifts and talents. Are they being nurtured? In our Super Woman ways, we try desperately to create Super Offspring, often at the expense of nurturing their true gifts. There is so much competition in today's world to have well-rounded kids. They know a little bit about a lot of things, but each child has a special talent. I challenge you to sit down with each child and discuss this with him or her. Kids get stressed out, too, and they may be relieved to have your blessing to cut down on some of their activities.

Home Time

Does your house stress you out? I don't mean your mortgage payment—who doesn't that stress out? I mean, when you walk through your front door, how do you feel? Are you happy to be home? What about when someone else shows up at your front door? Does just the sound of the UPS truck entering your driveway send you running outside before he can reach your door so he can't see inside your house? When a friend says, "We should get together soon" do you immediately reply, "Sure. Let's make it your house," because you're too embarrassed to have anyone over to yours?

Pam Young and Peggy Jones, two sisters who are self-proclaimed born slobs and authors of *Sidetracked Home Executives: From Pigpen to Paradise* (Warner, 2001), calls this CHAOS: Can't Have Anyone Over Syndrome. I love that, first of all because it's so creative, but secondly, because it's so true! The clutter creates too much embarrassment to entertain

115

friends and family. We get so stressed-out over the mess in our homes it makes us sick—physically and emotionally. It can be dangerous, too. If there was an emergency—let's say someone in your house cut themselves badly—could you clean it off in your kitchen sink right now? Or is it full of long over-due dirty dishes? Is there a clean towel handy? Could you grab your car keys and purse and be out the door in 30 seconds or less? Would there be enough gas in your vehicle to get there? When you got to the hospital, would your insurance cards and/or some form of money be in your purse? Would it be in a handy, reliable spot in your purse? Or would you have to stand there, pawing through the entire thing, saying, "I know it's in here, somewhere," while your patient, who really needs to be seen right away and is getting uglier by the second, has to sit there and wait while you find the appropriate documentation?

Emergency situations not withstanding, our average, day-to-day lives also suffer from our lack of disorganization and over abundance of clutter. One theory is that our perfectionism is what makes us slobs. I didn't understand this at first, because it seemed so opposite to me. Shouldn't a perfectionist be an obsessive neat-freak? But then I began thinking about how I am. I'm a perfectionist in certain areas of my life. If something is worth doing (as the old saying goes) it's worth doing well—or perfect. So when it came to housework, I wanted it done right...or not at all. And I wanted it all done, not just little chunks of it. Consequently, it didn't get done. Oh sure, the major things, like vacuuming, got done once a week. But there were almost always dirty dishes left over from the night before, because I was "too tired" to deal with them. The bathroom might go three or four weeks without a good cleaning. Dusting? Fuhgeddaboudit. And there was always laundry that just couldn't seem to make its way into the drawers and closets where it belonged. Then there was the clutter. It just seemed to grow out of nowhere. And the bigger the piles became, the less I had the time to deal with them. Was I sick of the mess? Sure. It totally stressed me out! I was a total SHE (Side-tracked Home Executive) with CHAOS. While I was working outside the home, I could keep a nice, neat desk at work, but when it came to home, who had the time? I certainly didn't think I did.

The first step for me came in changing my attitude, and acting upon my stressors (remember our steps in dealing with stress?). I had to accept that there was something I could do about the mess and take care of things that needed to be taken care of, even if I didn't like doing them. I figured since they had to be done, I might as well have a cheerful attitude about it. It's a choice. Either whine and complain about doing it, or do it and be happy. I figured I had a lot more to be thankful for than not, so I changed how I looked at even the most mundane chores.

A Coaching Moment

What necessary things in your life do you need to change your attitude about?

Before I give away any more of my secrets, though, let me fully convince you why you should take action and how your life is affected by your clutter.

It's costly. How many finance charges are incurred due to late payments? How many checks are bounced because we "don't have the time" to balance the checkbook? How many things come up "missing," so we buy a new one, only to discover months later that the original one was just buried underneath our piles of junk? This is all such a waste of money! Yeah. It might be just a few dollars here and there, but if you took the time to add up how much money you waste because of clutter, you'd be amazed!

It's stressful. We've already examined how stress can affect every system in our bodies. From contributing to heart disease to cancer to gastrointestinal problems, stress is a killer. But have you ever thought about where your personal stress comes from? Take a break from reading this for a moment, and look up from your book. What do your surroundings look like? How does it make you feel? When you walk into your house, are you happy to be there? Or does it just remind you of all the mess that still needs to be taken care of? Our homes should be a respite from the stress of life outside the home. Our homes should not be a major source of our stress. I don't care what kind of home you live in, whether it's a mobile home, an apartment, or a palace, it can still be taken care of and kept clean and clutter-free.

It's disrespectful of others' time. *Others time? How in the world does my mess affect someone else's time?* Simple. How many times a week are you late? Living in a disorganized mess is an almost automatic indicator that you will be late to many appointments. How can you be on time when you can't find shoes and keys and purse? Oh yeah, and your watch. *But I've got all these kids to get out the door, too.* We'll discuss in a minute some tips on how to get yourself (and your family) more organized, but let me just say this: being late, especially when you're consistently late, is like you saying that the other person's time is not as valuable as your own time.

It's dirty. When we have piles of clutter that just sit there, dust and dirt collect around and over it all. Then, since we don't want to move it to dust under it, we go around it (if at all), while the piles continue to grow. If the stuff is shoved underneath the bed and couch, we can't vacuum under them. If the kitchen sink is always piled high of dirty dishes, we can't clean it. If the counter is covered with piles of stuff, we can't clean that either, let alone cook on it.

It's time-consuming. How many times have you walked out your door and arrived to your destination, only to realize you forgot something—something major? I know I've done this. I've promised a friend I would let her borrow something, and half-way to her house, I realized I'd forgotten to bring what I promised I would let her borrow. So then I have to turn around and go back to my house to grab it. What a waste of time! Not to mention, that then I'm late getting to her house! How much time do you waste looking for things? What are your mornings like? There's an orange juice commercial that first shows (in black and white) a scene of more simple times. The kids make their beds in the morning, a hot breakfast is waiting for them when they come down to the kitchen, and they've got plenty of time to eat. Then the T.V. tells you to "get real" and it becomes colored, with a frantic family trying to gulp down OJ and get out the door. It stresses me out just watching it! Which scene best depicts your morning? The dishonest thing about this commercial is that it makes it seem as though the first scenario is impossible. Well I'm here to tell you, it's not! When your house isn't a cluttered mess and you're halfway organized and plan ahead, you can actually have enjoyable mornings! Which is a good segue for our next section...

Tips For Cleaning Up Your Act

There is so much that can be said on this topic, of course, that whole books are written on the subject. If you'd like to read more about getting the clutter out of your house and schedule, check out the "Good Reads" section at the end of this book. For now, though, I'd like to highlight some important points that have helped me clean up my act. Fine-tune and tailor these tactics to fit your own personality and cut down on clutter in your home, including the time-sucking elements that keep you running on a treadmill, never getting anywhere. If it makes you feel any better, I'm still working at it. Once a clutter-bug, always a clutter-bug at heart...to a certain extent. But you can break free from clutter bondage. It's hard work, but I'm here to tell you, you won't even believe the change in yourself and your family. It is so worth it! Without further ado...

De-clutter first. Do not, I repeat, do not go out and buy a bunch of storage containers—yet. I know—it's such an "in" thing to have a nice neat arrangement of storage apparatus. It makes it look as if you're really organized. But if you go and buy a bunch of containers, you're not going to know what you really need, since the first step in cleaning up should be to get rid of the extra junk first. Storing all the clutter pretty much defeats your purpose. Doesn't it? So, de-clutter first, store later.

Work in small chunks of time. Many of us will fare better if we set aside a small amount of time each day dedicated to de-cluttering. Part of our problem has been that we're waiting until we have a free day to do it all. But that day never seems to arrive. So pencil in 15 or 20 minutes of de-cluttering time each day to begin sifting out the clutters.

Do it now. Stop contributing to the current clutter. When you pick up the mail, go through it then. Do not add it to the pile. Groceries? Put them all away. Kids schoolwork? Toss it, file it, or hang it. Dishes? Do them up after each meal. Laundry? Put it right away after folding it.

Make it a habit/routine. Make cleaning up your act a habit. This means you must do it regularly and consistently which also means you must think rather than live subconsciously.

Don't wait until it looks dirty. Do you wait to dust until there's an inch of dirt covering everything and the dust bunnies come hopping out from underneath the beds and tables all on their own? Does the bathroom not get cleaned until mildew is hanging from the ceiling and the bathtub requires a jackhammer to get off the build-up? I used to hate to dust, so I would let about three months or so go between dustings. Oh yeah! Talk about dust bunnies. We had many generations of them living in our house (you know how quickly those rabbits multiply!). And then it was such a chore when I finally did do it, that I grumbled (not to mention sneezed and wheezed) the whole time. Now our house gets a quick dusting about three or four times a week. The awesome thing about doing these chores regularly is that, because it's not so dirty, it doesn't take as long to clean. You don't have to devote your entire Saturday to housework. If you devote a few minutes each day to cleanup, you stay on top of everything and your house is always visitor-ready—even if it's just the UPS guy.

Get the right equipment. Part of what has made dusting more enjoyable for me is simply having the right tools for the job. The dusting cloths they make nowadays are a fabulous invention. It's especially nice with allergies, since the dust sticks to them, and doesn't fly off everywhere—and no messy spray to deal with. Ditto for the bathroom and floors. The disinfectant wipes and pre-moistened cleaning pads make for quick and easy clean-up.

Designate certain days for certain activities. In our house, Mondays, Wednesdays, and Fridays are dusting days. The bathrooms get a quick wipe-down everyday (yes, I said everyday!). The main living areas of the house are given a quick vacuuming almost every day. At least one load of laundry is done each day and on Saturday the bathrooms get a more thorough cleaning. By designating days, it makes it much easier to make it a habit. Think back to your grandmother. How did she get all her chores done? Chances are, days were designated for specific activities: one day was laundry day, one day was errand and shopping day, one day was bread-baking day, etc. But don't use my schedule as your model. Only you can determine how often chores need to be done. Decide what works for you and your household.

Delegate. Besides having the right tools, dusting has also become more enjoyable for me, because I don't always do it! Each of my sons is assigned different chores for the week (and paid for doing them), including dusting, cleaning the bathrooms, dry dusting the floors, sweeping the deck, washing windows, and helping out with laundry (and if you have daughters, I'll be taking applications for their wives in about 15 years!). Getting your kids involved (while they may complain about it) helps to instill a good work ethic, as well as instilling a feeling of belonging—you're a family unit, a team, and one that should all work together.

Plan ahead. If you've read through the book to this point, the idea of making a plan is nothing earth-shattering. Too many of us take life as it comes, never really thinking ahead far enough to prepare for anything. As an example, tell me what you're having for dinner two nights from now. Let me guess—haven't thought that far into the week, have you? Let me take another stab—when you decide that morning (or afternoon) what you'll have, you'll run to the store to get the necessary ingredients (or pick it up at the drive-through, since you didn't plan supper until suppertime, and didn't have time to cook anything). Having a plan applies to almost every area of our lives, including home and schedule de-cluttering. Plan out your week, including what each day will include, right down to what chores need to be accomplished that day and what you're planning for meals. Write it down. Eventually, after it all becomes a true habit, you won't need to write out everything— it will come more naturally.

Make a list. A written list should be a part of your plan. It always feels good to check things off, giving you a feeling of accomplishment. It also helps you organize your day. If you need to, write the list down on a time schedule, allotting different amounts of time for each activity. Be realistic, though.

If you need to run errands, and you know you'll hit highway construction on the way, be sure to give yourself enough time.

A Coaching Moment

Where do you need to begin today to clean up your act? Your house? Your schedule? Choose one and begin to tackle it one step at a time.

For You Creative, Spontaneous Types...

If you're thinking this would never work for me. I can't live by routines and schedules. I need my freedom. Let me ask you something. Do you feel free surrounded by a mess? Do you feel free when you can't walk through your home without stepping on toys or clothes or old food, or stubbing your foot on something because it's not where it belongs? Do you feel safe walking through your house barefoot, unworried you'll step on something and cut your foot? Do you feel free when you open your drawers and there is nothing to wear because the laundry hasn't been done? Do your creative juices really flow, knowing that you should be cleaning up the pigpen you call home? I know for myself, as a writer, I can have a very pressing deadline, and what do I do when I should be writing? De-clutter! I can't stand to try to work in the middle of a mess anymore. I know I should be working, but I need to clear the area so that I can think clearly—clearing the mess also clears my brain. Other people have said the same thing. Once they began to get into flexible routines and consistent habits, they actually felt more creative and were able to work in a more relaxed environment. So give it a try. You may find that you can be even more spontaneous and actually enjoy life more knowing you have a clean, uncluttered home waiting for you.

Stepping Stones

- Learning to de-clutter your schedule is imperative to living a life of wellness.
- Follow the process for change when de-cluttering: desire, choose, plan, and act.
- Perfectionist, all-or-nothing attitudes may be holding you captive in your own home.
- Clutter is costly, stressful, disrespectful, dirty, and time consuming.
- Following a flexible routine and de-cluttering will free your creative juices and allow you to be even more spontaneous—without the guilt.

CHAPTER NINE

Creating A Plan To Dump Your Garbage

Now that you've made a decision to cross the bridge and dump that old chaos, disorganization and "fluffy" baggage, there's one thing you'll need to do before you act—have a plan. Remember—desire, choose, plan, act. So many of us float through life aimlessly, trying this and that, going here and there, never really stopping to think about what we're actually doing, but always hoping that whatever it is, it'll work. As an example…you've got ten seconds to tell me what you had to eat yesterday. Hurry! Time's a wastin'! You see? It's hard, isn't it, to even recall what we ate just 24 hours ago. This is because we shove things into our mouths—whatever is available and within arm's reach—without even thinking about what it is we're doing. I call this subconscious eating (or unconscious eating—take your pick!). We do this with many things in our lives. For instance, we allow (or force) our kids to sign up for everything available to them—soccer, karate, swimming, art lessons, drama, dance, and any other club you can think of—without even considering the effects of having schedules so crammed they can't breathe. (Not to mention what it's doing to the whole family's health and dynamics).

Ditto for our own schedules. How many committees do you currently belong to? What groups are you leading, simply because "no one else will do it" or because you'd feel too guilty if you turned them down? How many extra projects do you take on at work, regardless of whether or not you've got the time and energy (you'll just bring the work home if you can't get it done at the office—your family will understand, right?) either because you feel obligated to or because "no one else will do it?" How many evenings are you spending at home, winding down from the day and preparing your body for rest? How many evenings is the whole family at home together? If you're like most families, not too many.

> When we fill our lives with too much 'fluff' it appears full from the outside, but the inside really has no substance—or sustenance.

You see, so much of our lives is spent just crossing tasks off the list—either literally or in our minds. Am I against making a "to-do" list? Absolutely not! If you read the previous chapter, you know that I feel it's an important organizational tool. But having a plan, based on your purpose, is way more than just having a list. Having a plan includes actually taking the time to think through and decide how you will live and what you will include in your life. What is really important to you? What is just "fluff?" When we fill our lives with too much "fluff," it appears full from the outside, but the inside really has no substance—or sustenance. The "fullness" is really just comprised of meaningless busyness that keeps us going in a million different directions. How can we possibly give our best when we're spread so thin others can see right through us? We can't!

Let's examine four steps of planning more closely.

A Coaching Moment

What in your life has been holding you back from being the woman you were created to be?

STEP ONE: **The first part of your plan should entail a little cognitive work.** Take a deep look at your life and where it's headed. Are you spinning your wheels, getting nowhere in particular? Are you content with where you're at right now? I'm not just talking career. Even if you're a stay-at-home mom, have you made peace with your current calling? It took me years to accept my role as mother and being at home. I was always looking for something else, like I couldn't possibly be satisfied and fulfilled with changing diapers, nursing nonstop, being peed, pooped, and spit on (sometimes all at once!), dealing with whiney, bickering children (sounds like some adults I know!), spending all day in the kitchen trying to satisfy everyone's picky tastes…talk about lowly! But it wasn't until I finally did accept my calling and choose to be happy doing it, that God allowed one of my desires to actually materialize—writing. It was like I sort of had to show Him I could handle what He had given me—not just physically carrying out my duties, but pouring my heart into it, as well—before He could trust me with something more.

Where are you right now? What is really just "fluff," creating unnecessary busyness, and what do you really care about? This all goes right back to living life on purpose, rather than by accident. People who live their lives on purpose don't have fluffy lives—lives filled with unnecessary, meaningless things.

A Coaching Moment

Is your life headed in the direction it should be to fulfill your purpose in life? Or are you holding onto others' expectations? What do you need to do to dump this perception and begin living your life according to your purpose—rather than according to what others think it should be?

STEP TWO: To help you determine what's fluff and what's meaningful, make a chart with three columns.
"Meaningful," "Necessary," and "Fluff," and start listing everything you do in one of the three columns. The necessary things are the things we talked about before —things we may or may not enjoy doing, but things that need to be done. Meaningful items are things that, while not seemingly necessary, add meaning to your life (and therefore, in the end, are, in fact, necessary). Include things that, if you had the time, you'd like to do. Fluff…well, you know what that is now. Once you've done this, take a look at what you've got. Examine the columns closely. Are the "Necessary" things you've included all really necessary? Are any of them really "fluff" in disguise?

Sometimes, things we think are mandatory really aren't. Sometimes, they're things other people think should be mandatory in our lives. If some things are left up in the air as to which category they should go into, try talking about them to someone, like your spouse or a close friend. Having someone to discuss your priorities with can help you gain proper perspective.

STEP THREE: In addition to creating your chart, write down how long you do each listed item during an average week.
Keep track of your time spent as you go through your week.

At the end of the week, evaluate your findings. You may be amazed at how much time you spend doing certain tasks! Compare your weekly analysis and your list. How do they mesh together? Are you spending a lot of time on "fluff?" How much time are you spending doing meaningful things? Are the necessary things eating up a lot of your time? Sounds like you could use a plan!

A Coaching Moment
What in your life is eating up your time, but not contributing to your purpose? What will you do about it?

STEP FOUR: **The next step of planning is to make your game plan.** Which items on your list of categories will help you meet your purpose? Probably not many of the "fluffy" things, right? Now you need to decide if you're going to keep the "fluff," or get rid of it. If you're going to keep it, then you'll need to decide how it all fits into a lifestyle of wellness (remember…you've made the decision to change!) and how you're going to make it work. If you're going to get rid of it, you'll need to plan out how to do that. Is there a project you need to finish before handing in your resignation? Are elections coming up for the next board members that you need to bow out of? Do you need to make a decision to just say "no thanks" the next time a big project is offered to you? Do you need to do something different about your job? Quit? Go part-time? Job share? Pick a job closer to home? Work from home? Start your own business? There really are many options, but you have to actually investigate them—and who's got the time for that? However, if you don't take the time, you're going to be stuck where you are. Is that a viable option at this point in your life? Will that contribute to you living a life of wellness?

You'll also want to make up a plan for those things you listed under "Necessary" and "Meaningful." Why? Because while it may be necessary, it doesn't necessarily mean you're doing it in a way that is conducive to living well. As an example, let's go back to grocery shopping. How many times a week do you find yourself inhabiting the supermarket? I'm not talking about stopping to buy milk. I'm talking, you decide that morning what you're having for dinner and go to the store to pick up what you need for that meal—and this happens several times a week. Talk about a waste of time! If you find yourself in this situation, what can you do to gain that time back? For starters, how about pre-planning your meals—before you go shopping? For ease of planning, how about designating each night of the week as a particular type of food? For instance, Monday is stir-fry night, Tuesday is roast night, Wednesday is pasta night, Thursday is breakfast night (we usually have breakfast foods, like waffles or pancakes with the fixings, for supper once a week!), Friday is surprise night (might be leftover night, or let members of your family decide each week what they want…), Saturday is soup or stew and bread night, and Sunday is free-for-all (we all deserve a day off!). If you like to eat out one night a week, designate that, too. This makes meal planning a cinch, as you just have to find recipes that fit into a particular category. Check out the "Good Reads" section for cookbooks that come with shopping lists.

Designate a day for shopping and pencil it into your schedule, treating it like an appointment you have to keep. Sometime prior to heading out the door on shopping day, make a list of the things you need—or a list of things you don't need.

I know we tend to buy the same basic things each week, so noting what I don't need that week or what special ingredients I need for a recipe makes more sense for us, rather than writing down everything we need. Check out the store's sales flyer for that week. If you use coupons, take out the ones you'll need for that day. Once there, shop for the whole week. Yeah, you may end up going back for milk later in the week. Not all of us have space to store several gallons at a time in our refrigerator, but that's to be expected. The real time-waster is going to the store multiple times in a week to do "mini" shopping.

A Coaching Moment
How can you more wisely organize your time?

This is just one example. You can apply this type of thinking to many things in your life. The four main keys under "dumping your garbage" include:
1. Establishing your purpose.
2. Determining what things in your life fit your purpose and eliminating those that don't fit.
3. Preparing for those things you're building your life around.
4. Establishing routines.

You will be amazed at how much time you "gain" in a day when you put these principles into place.

Ready, Set...Go!
Okay, so you really want to change and live a life of wellness. You've made the decision to do so, and you've got your plan in place. What's left? Borrowing from a well-known shoe

company, "Just do it!" The hardest part is over. Now it's time to go for it!

The key here is to make your change a habit. To do that, you need to commit to doing it consistently and routinely. Decide how often this new change needs to be done—daily, weekly, monthly. Schedule your budding new habit into your planner—not with a pencil, but with a pen! Remember—treat it like an appointment that cannot be broken. Schedule other things around your appointment, rather than scheduling it around everything else. If you follow the latter case, you will rarely end up making this new change a habit.

> Another idea for letting go of the past pain is to burn it. Literally. Write each item you've been holding onto on a separate piece of paper, then set them ablaze. While you're doing this, pray, meditate, and make a commitment to this new journey.

This all ties back into the other three stages, because you need the desire, you need to make a choice to continue doing it, and you need to plan ahead—and sometimes re-evaluate your plan. As you can see, while each step has a separate identity, they're all part of a much larger whole. We'll talk more specifically about how to move ahead and put your plan into action in upcoming chapters.

So now do you understand the kind of journey you're on? If you have any old baggage that needs to be thrown out, I encourage you to visit the landfill and dump it. You simply cannot begin a new journey carrying all that old baggage. What I often do is envision wrapping it all up and tossing the package upward. I figure He can deal with it much better than I can. If I choose to hold on to it, it becomes so heavy that the burden is too much to bear. Then it begins to affect other areas of my life. The sad irony is, the more you hold on to, the more you collect. And the baggage you carry may seem like a nice cushy wall of protection, but it will become your destruction. No one can live a life of wellness holding on to past hurts, fears, bitterness, hate, unforgiveness—you name it. Get rid of it.

Now are you ready to take the keys? Then let's go! In the following chapters, we're going to look at various aspects of living a life of wellness. Each one is a bridge within our journey. My hope is that this begins a lifelong process for you in becoming the woman you were created to be.

Stepping Stones

- Living a life of disorganization and "fluff" will not lead you in a direction of wellness.
- Take a look at your life and where it's headed.
- Decide what in your life is necessary, what is meaningful and what is fluff.
- Track your time and calculate how much time is spent doing the three different types of activities.
- Create a plan and establish routines to eliminate time-wasters.

PART THREE

Making Sense of What's Ahead

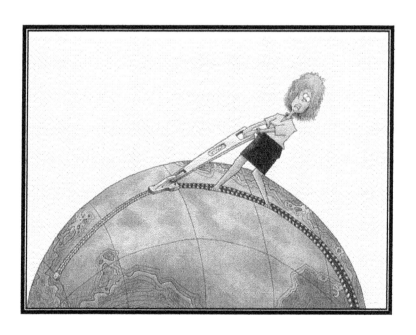

CHAPTER TEN

Brick Walls, Stone Fences, and Other Annoying Obstacles

(plus how to leap over them without tripping and falling flat on your face!)

No matter how dedicated or diligent you are in changing your habits and moving forward with your journey to wellness, you will inevitably walk, run, or at times, simply fall into obstacles along the way. Sometimes these obstacles are bumps in the road, other times they'll be aggravating potholes that take the air out of your tires. At one time or another, you'll have to cross a river—with no bridge in sight, hike a steep mountain—with no foreseeable end, and scale a rocky cliff—with no one around to help with the climbing gear. Before you think, "What's the use?" keep reading! With a little planning and a lot of prayer, you will get through setbacks, stand back on your feet (on dry, flat ground!), and continue moving forward.

Set backs or Failures?

Any sort of coach training, be it lifestyle, business, or wellness, involves a lot of education on human behavior and positive thinking. Part of a coach's job, after all, is to cheer her client on. As a coach, I don't ever want a client to think she's a failure and not worth the effort. I don't want a client to give up because she hasn't met her goals. In coaching, there is no failure, only setbacks.

Failure has gotten a really bum rap. These days it's seen as a very negative thing. If we fail, we lose. The end. Kaput. Setbacks, on the other hand, imply that we've just met one of those bumps in the road, but will get through it and move on. I feel, however, that to totally ignore our failures is to be dishonest to ourselves. There are times when we do flat out fail. For instance, if I set a deadline to finish this book and don't meet it, is it just a failure…or a setback? The book isn't a failure (or at least I hope not!), and I don't consider myself a failure. Accepting and learning from failure, doesn't make you a failure. I can still work on finishing it and getting it out. But I did fail to meet my deadline. That's honesty. That's reality. To say that I'm just experiencing a setback is an excuse. It's that balance thing again. While I certainly believe in looking at the positive, that needs to be balanced with taking a peek at reality, as well.

I also don't believe that failure is always negative. Many professional athletes take failure and turn it into energy. Entrepreneurs take a failed

> It's when you take your failure and turn it inside-out—examine it, take it apart, get down and dirty with it, and most of all, learn from it—that you can create something positive from a negative experience.

business deal and turn it into success. It's when you take your failure and turn it inside-out—examine it, take it apart, get down and dirty with it, and most of all, learn from it—that you can create something positive from a negative experience.

In her book, *Optimal Thinking: How to be Your Best Self* (Wiley, 2002), Rosalene Glickman, Ph.D. explains that optimal thinking goes beyond just positive thinking. Optimal thinking, she says, is optimal realism—it is not optimism. In other words, optimal thinking is that balance between thinking positively and considering the negative. Think of it as neutral thinking. Let's use a topic that was really hot a few years ago: Y2K. Remember that? Doomsday! Right? As we know now, the hype was just that—hype. But what end of the see saw were you on? Were you one of the ones that stockpiled food and ammunition? Did you go and trade your money for gold? Did you buy chickens and a cow so you'd have meat, milk, and eggs? Or were you a total unbeliever, who didn't do a thing to prepare for the "just in case?" You were going to party and welcome in the New Year (I'm skirting the when-the-millennium-really-started issue here!) with the same carefree attitude you had every previous year. You figured if it's going to happen, it's going to happen, and no amount of preparation

---

Human Behavior Specialists have come up with the Stages of Change, scientifically referred to as The Transtheoretical Approach for Change—(say that five times fast!). This progressive order of readiness helps us determine where we are in our readiness to change a habit.

---

would help. Or maybe you were like most people. While you didn't panic, you did make sure you had enough food and water for about a week. You may have had a transistor radio and some extra batteries. You didn't stick your head in the sand, but you didn't run around screaming, "The sky is falling!" for a year beforehand, either. That's optimal thinking!

You weighed in on both the pros and cons, and found a healthy balance between the two. Thinking too positively during that time could have gotten you into trouble, had something happened. Those of you who thought too negatively, well, I hope you donated all that canned food to the food bank!

Sometimes failure allows us to take an honest look at what we're doing. Sometimes it opens our eyes to the fact that we're not quite ready to begin this newest leg of our journey. At times, we'll need to pitch a tent and stay for a while, camp out. We need to focus on "the now" rather than set our sites for "the then." Sometimes we need to get reacquainted with ourselves before moving ahead with more change. And that's okay. This also gives us time to plan and prepare for the next change coming our way. It's during these times that we often learn more about ourselves and gain a greater understanding of who we are—and come out feeling better about ourselves in the process, and ready and refreshed to continue on with our journey.

A Coaching Moment

Which end of the spectrum have you been placing too much emphasis on regarding various situations or activities in your life? What have you been thinking too positively or too negatively about? This type of thought creates unrealism, and doesn't allow you to create an optimal environment for growth. List out the pros and cons of a situation or habit, and weigh them against each other. Find a balanced solution to the situation and be the best you can be!

In a Nutshell,
The Stages of Change Are:

Pre-contemplation: You're not really thinking about change at this point, because you either think you can't change (lack of self-confidence) or just flat out won't, because you don't see a reason to (stubbornness or naiveté). If you think you can't change a behavior, analyze the reasons behind your feelings. If you just don't want to, look into the behavior more, and its implications on your health. Sometimes what just seems like a little bad habit can have huge health consequences.

Contemplation: At this point, you're thinking you might change a behavior in the future—usually within six months or so. It's easy to get stuck in this stage, so pull out the tire chains and do more research, if necessary, about the health implications of holding onto this behavior. Weigh its pros and cons. Think about small steps you can take to begin chipping away at changing it.

Preparation: By now, you're thinking I will change this behavior in the very near future—usually within the next month or so (can you feel the climax building?!). It's important at this stage to prepare and formalize your plan of attack. Get the necessary tools in place that will contribute to your success. List out potential obstacles you're likely to encounter and their possible solutions. Strategize! Put on your armor, baby, it's time to rock 'n roll!

Action: Finally, you're ready to put some action into your plan! This stage usually lasts up to six months or so. During this phase, you're working on actually changing a habit—either replacing an unhealthy habit with a healthier one, adding a healthy habit, or kicking an unhealthy one all together. Don't be surprised if you slip back into old habits now and then during this stage. That's where your planning comes in, and why you should not skip the preparation stage. Work on continually refining your strategies for success to keep yourself on track.

Maintenance: Whew! You made it! You've established a new, healthy habit! Congratulations! Now what? You keep on, keeping on, that's what—and enjoy your life even more as the new, healthier you. Even at this point, however, it's easy to relapse back into old ways. Rather than wallowing in self-pity, go back to the preparation phase and lay out your plan again. What in your original plan worked? What didn't? Life is constantly evolving—chances are, your plan needs a little updating. Adapt it to where you are now. Because you have already succeeded at changing this habit in the past, you will most likely move through this leg of the journey with a little more ease than the first time through.

One Little, Two Little, Three Little Obstacles...

As I said a few pages back, no matter how dedicated you are to your plan, you will hit obstacles (sometimes, they'll even try to run you flat over!). The number of obstacles you run into has nothing to do with your diligence to your changes. You may go through times when there's an obstacle waiting around every bend. This doesn't

> "Obstacles often are not personal attacks; they are muscle builders."
> —Anne Wilson Schaef

mean you're doing something wrong. How you handle the obstacles, however, will have everything to do with your success.

Susan Cantwell does an excellent job describing various kinds of obstacles we face in her book, *Mind Over Matter: Personal Choices for a Lifetime of Fitness* (Stoddart, 1999). She also, by the way, goes into more detail about that Transtheoretical Approach for Change model, in case you're interested! Cantwell differentiates obstacles from other bumps in the road, so for matter of simplification, let's use the umbrella term, roadblocks. There are three different kinds of roadblocks: barriers, obstacles, and excuses. I know you're anxious to get to that last one, so let's start with barriers (I have to keep your attention somehow!).

"A barrier," says Cantwell, "is an unpreventable event or circumstance that hinders our plans or actions." These are often last-minute situations that pop up—your child gets sent home from school because he inadvertently redesigned the classroom color scheme due to a stomach bug. When the school nurse called, you were on your way out the door to the gym, but instead, now have to go pick up your heaving honey and spend the rest of the day dodging barf buckets. Here's another example—your husband calls at the last minute to say he needs to work late. He usually watches the kids while you workout. A barrier is just one of those things that you need to accept and work around. Sometimes, the last-minute or unexpected will totally prevent you from accomplishing your goal. And illness, for instance, can totally derail us from meeting our goals during that time (of illness).

Cantwell describes an obstacle as "a foreseeable event or circumstance that impedes our plans or actions." A work schedule could fall into this category. You know ahead of time what it is—whether it's yours or your husband's—and you work with that to create your plan. This will usually involve re-arranging things in your schedule that can be changed.

Sometimes, what first looks like a barrier, if given enough thought, can become an obstacle. Remember, barriers stop you in your tracks—you can't do anything about them. But with an obstacle, there are choices and solutions. Let's look at the barrier example where your husband calls last-minute to say he can't be there to watch the kids while you go to your exercise class. Now what? Are there other options? Could you workout at home with an exercise video? Could you take all the kids and go for a walk? Could you go outside and play active games with the kids? Do you have some dumbbells at home you could use? A treadmill or bike? Is there a neighbor or friend who could watch them for that short time? Perhaps these options would work, but it depends on the ages of your kids and the time of day. If it's suppertime, it wouldn't be a very fruitful workout if they need to eat. Would it? Or if it's after suppertime, and your husband normally gets them ready for bed, trying to workout with cranky, tired kids would just get you more stressed out. We'll talk in a minute about how to ask yourself powerful questions to determine powerful solutions to your barriers and obstacles.

The third and final roadblock (and I know you've been waiting for this one!) is just what it says it is: an excuse. According to Cantwell, an excuse is "an event or circumstance, foreseeable or unforeseeable, that with planning, could be overcome." Trying to squeeze ourselves into molds we don't fit into encourages the creation of excuses. Because we know we can't fit into some mold we think we should be fitting into, we find one excuse after another not to initiate or stick with healthy changes. Once we break out of this mindset, we find ourselves tailoring our lives to who we are and what fits us, rather than trying to squeeze into molds that were never meant for us in the first place. At last, we find joy!

A Coaching Moment

Got your journal handy? Make three columns: barriers, obstacles, excuses. Begin placing healthy-living barriers, obstacles, and excuses that you encounter under each column. It's important to be honest and admit your excuses. Once you've finished that, take each obstacle and come up with possible solutions for them. Then throw out all those excuses!

How To Hurdle Obstacles With Grace

You're at a party, and end up sitting next to someone you don't really know, who seemingly isn't interested in carrying on a conversation with you, and answers your questions with the shortest possible replies. The whole time you're thinking, Someone rescue me!

Possible solutions?

A. Nonchalantly (and accidentally, of course!) drop your drink into your lap and immediately excuse yourself to the restroom.

B. Use the old, "Oh! I haven't seen so-and-so for ages!" exclamation (even if you have no idea who the other person is or if it's actually your best friend). Tell your duddy party buddy how nice it was to meet them, quickly excuse yourself, and run!

C. Use powerful questions to get the other person to open up and relax.

While you may have tried any and all of these solutions at one time or another, the last option is the best (and most polite!) since many times, it's not just the other person who causes this plight. When it feels like you're pulling teeth trying to get the other person to talk, maybe it's because you're not asking the right questions. This same idea can be applied to conversations with ourselves, too (What? Don't you talk to yourself?), and is imperative when you're trying to find solutions and strategize on overcoming obstacles.

Asking powerful questions begins with minimizing the use of closed ended questions. You know, the ones that require a one-word reply. "Do I want to workout today?" requires a simple yes or no answer (and what's your most likely

> Powerful questions produce powerful responses, which in turn, produce powerful solutions.

answer?). "What can I do to ensure I get my workout in today?" demands a more detailed response. It makes you think about your schedule and how you can fit your workout into your day. It causes you to plan ahead and strategize solutions to any potential or known obstacles. Powerful questions produce powerful responses, which in turn, produce powerful solutions.

Most powerful questions begin with what and how. Beginning your questions with what and how invokes action-oriented, practical solutions. "How can I plan my meals out better?" makes you think about hands-on, practical solutions to better meal planning.

You can also use "why" questions; however, doing so tends to encourage emotional responses rather than hands-on ones. For instance, "Why can't I seem to get my workout in?" opens the way for the old, "because I just don't feel like it" excuse. "Why do I always seem to overeat?" opens the conversation to "because I just can't control myself." If used inappropriately, "why" questions can be power sapping, rather than powerful.

There are times, however, when a "why" question is appropriate—usually after you've asked yourself the "what" and "how" questions and still haven't seen success. "Why do I always overeat?" can also lend itself to digging deeper into emotional eating. "Why can't I seem to get my workout in?" could make you think about how you feel about your body, going to the gym, and your fitness vision.

> If used inappropriately, "why" questions can be power sapping, rather than powerful.

When used appropriately, asking the "why" questions will take you back a step, but will ultimately allow you to move forward in your journey—as opposed to spinning your wheels and not going anywhere! For instance, with the workout question, you may uncover that you feel embarrassed working out at the gym with other women who are in much better shape. So you avoid going. You took a step back to admit this, and now you can ask yourself the "how" and "what" questions to move yourself forward again. In this case, a couple of possibilities, depending on which direction you wanted to take, would be, "What are some options to working out at the gym?" or "While I feel embarrassed, what do I feel the other members think about me being there?" The answer to the first question could be a number of things. You could workout at home with videos, stationary equipment, and weights. You could do outdoor activities. You could join a women-only gym. The answer to the second question will be more subjective, but it can help put things into perspective. The probable answer would be that the other members think it's great that you're there taking care of yourself. Some of them have, at one point, been where you are now, and so they empathize with you, and are cheering you on (even if you don't realize it). A good way to answer questions like this is to turn the table: if it were you who was very fit, and an unfit member worked out next to you, what would you be thinking? Wouldn't you be routing them on, thinking that it's great they're there?

A Coaching Moment

Is there one area where you can't seem to move forward? Write it down. Now ask yourself powerful questions beginning with what and how. Come up with practical, hands-on solutions to getting over this hurdle.

Stepping Stones

- Take your failure, turn it inside-out, and create something positive from it.
- Find a realistic balance between being totally pessimistic and totally optimistic.
- Determine which stage of change you're in for a particular habit and decide to move forward.
- Work around the barriers, hurdle the obstacles, and burn the excuses!

- You will most likely experience setbacks in your progress—use powerful questions to avoid making a setback permanent.
- Powerful questions produce powerful responses, which in turn, produce powerful solutions.
- Begin powerful questions with how and what first, to strategize practical, hands-on solutions.
- If the "how" and "what" questions don't result in success, use the "why" questions to dig deeper.
- Don't get stuck on "why" questions—use them to take a step back and then move forward with action questions.

CHAPTER ELEVEN

Putting Your Plan Together

We often hear the phrase "follow your dreams." What are *your* dreams? Don't skim this—really think about it. We've all had dreams at one point or another. But life takes over and our dreams get stuffed into some back closet, waiting for a time when we've got just that—more time. Let me tell you something—we'll never have as much time as we'd like! There will always be "urgent" stuff—not truly urgent, but urgent, because that's how most of us live our lives—on adrenaline and caffeine, creating last-minute chaos, because we haven't planned ahead.

Stop for a moment and think back to a time in your life when you had dreams. What were they? If you could incorporate healthy changes into your life, along with a dream or two, what would life look like five years from now?

> "Picture yourself in your mind's eye as having already achieved this goal. See yourself doing the things you'll be doing when you've reached your goal." - Earl Nightingale

This is the first part of your plan—your "Wellness Vision." It's upon this Wellness Vision—along with a couple other things—that your plan will be built.

A Coaching Moment

Take a few minutes to seriously consider where you'd like to be five years from now. Sometimes it helps to get yourself into a quiet place, close your eyes, and picture yourself in your mind's eye to get a good visual idea of your vision. Write your Wellness Vision down using the most creative language you can muster.

Now I want you to think about your purpose in life. We discussed this in Chapter 8 when we discussed "de-fluffing" our schedules. What do you feel your purpose—or mission—is? What are your passions? Usually, our purpose and passions overlap. If you have a difficult time honing in on your purpose in life, I recommend you take a pit stop and go through at least one of several books, listed in the back of this book. One I highly recommend is *Passion on Purpose: Discovering and Pursuing a Life that Matters Most* by Deborah Newman, Ph.D. I like this one, because it's written for women by a woman. You cannot continue to flounder your way through life, and live life with any sort of purpose. It's difficult to live life by accident and achieve anything of worth—it's impossible to live your purpose this way. You must stop living life by accident and begin to live life on purpose if you are to live a life in wellness!

Begin by writing down what you think your purpose, or mission in life, is. You may have one main purpose or you may have a list. Your purpose may change from one season of your life to another. If you have small children, your main purpose at this time, may be to raise them. If this is the case, consider your passions, gifts, and talents, and how you think God may want you to use them now and in the future. Start writing!

151

When you get done, either leave this in list form (or as a sentence if that's all you came up with, in which case, that's okay!), or put it into a more readable format—the choice is yours. In any event, you have now laid out your personal mission statement, which now needs a title. Since this is your own statement, use your name in the title: "Mary's Personal Mission Statement" or "Mary's Life on Purpose Statement" or how about "Mary's Passion on Purpose Statement." Whatever you choose as your title, include the date you wrote it, as well. Sometimes, as we go further on our journey, our mission in life becomes more and more clear to us. It's cool to be able to look back and see how far we've come, how much we've grown.

A Coaching Moment

What do you feel you were put on this planet to do? What's your purpose in life? We all have a reason for being put on this earth—none less important than anyone else's. Write your Mission Statement down and then compare it to your Wellness Vision. Do the two mesh together? Is your Wellness Vision realistic? Make sure your vision doesn't include unrealistic ideals—like wanting a super model body on your 4' 9" frame!

The next step in your journey is to create and write out your goals. It's pretty amazing to see how, throughout history, many

> "Without goals, and plans to reach them, you are like a ship that has set sail with no destination." —Fizhugh Dodson

great people talk about goal-setting and its necessity to one's accomplishments.

Setting goals helps you determine where you're going and your focus each step of the way. As I've said throughout this book, you cannot just flounder your way through life and expect to live your purpose and meet your goals. And I've got research to back me up. Studies show that when goal-setting is included in participants' tool boxes for behavioral change, they are much more likely to succeed and create new, healthier habits.

That sounds great in theory and for the lab, you say, *but this is real life!*

"Goal setting works!" exclaims MaryAnn Koopmann, one of my Women in Wellness™ clients (and no, I did not pay or otherwise bribe her into saying that!). "Goal-setting has helped me succeed in my wellness plan because I set the goals myself to fit my needs and lifestyle with the help of my coach. It gives me direction and guides me to where I want to be. It gives me drive to keep myself in touch with what I need to do to succeed. I get pleasure when I can meet or beat them. A sense of accomplishment when I meet my goals only makes me thrive for more."

> According to Margaret Moore, CEO of Wellcoaches™, setting goals. . .
>
> . . . forces us to think about our motivators, the pros and cons of changing behaviors, and develop strategies for overcoming our obstacles
>
> . . . allows us to determine and measure success
>
> . . . helps us establish baselines so that we can monitor and celebrate how far we've come

Goal-setting, says MaryAnn, has been a big key in her success so far. "Everyone needs goals whether they are small or large. It will give you something to strive for. When I meet my goals for the week, it gives me a sense of completeness and I know I did my best. I push myself to do more than I do when I don't have any goals set for myself."

When setting your goals, it's important to have long-term and short-terms goals. Three months is a good time frame around which to build your long-term goals, since this is long enough to form new habits, but short enough to see the light at the end of the tunnel. If you set a long-term goal based on a year, it can become quite tedious to try to scrape your way to meet it. A year can seem like a lifetime, especially when trying to establish new habits. Once you have your three-month goals set, break them down, week-by-week as you go along, into short-term goals.

So what makes a "good" goal? One that is SMART! Goals should be Specific, Measurable, Action-oriented, Realistic, and Time-oriented.

> "A goal properly set is halfway reached."
> —Zig Ziglar

Specific: Your goals should be as specific and focused as possible. An example of a poorly worded goal is "to exercise regularly." While this certainly is a good goal in and of itself, it gives you nothing specific to shoot for. What kind of exercise are you talking about? Cardio? Strength training? Stretching? How often will you do it? Is there a certain time or frequency goal you need to include?

A better way to word this three-month goal would be something like, "to consistently do a cardio workout three times a week for 20 minutes each within my target heart rate zone." Just how specific you get depends on where you are in your journey to wellness. If you're a newbie, you may only need to set a goal, "to do two cardio workouts a week for 20 minutes each." It all depends on where you are now, and where you're headed.

Measurable: The goals you set should be measurable. In our examples above, you can easily measure the number of times you workout, the length of the workout, and your heart rate. Being able to measure the success of your progress takes away the subjectivity factor. You know what I mean! If you're trying to pay more attention to serving sizes, for instance, you could measure

One good word to keep in mind when you're setting goals is FITT. FITT stands for Frequency, Intensity, Time, and Type. While this acronym was designed specifically for fitness, you can also apply it to other goals—although you may not always use all the parts. For instance, you can set a nutrition goal to eat five fruits and vegetables five days a week. In this case, you've told the frequency (five days), time (or amount—five), and type (fruits and veggies). Just one tool to stick into your toolbox!

out your portion sizes...or you could just make an emotionally-filled, uneducated guess! I mean, after all, broken cookies and cleaning off the kids' plates don't count. Right? Measuring your goal-progress allows you to live consciously—as opposed to subconsciously (much better than *un*consciously, but still...). It doesn't allow room for self-sabotage—unless you just outright lie to yourself.

A Coaching Moment

I encourage my clients to keep a separate list of desires—things that may be immeasurable but are still goal-like. For instance, you may want to spend more time with your family or maybe you just want to laugh more. These aren't things you'll actually measure (unless some laugh-o-meter is invented in the near future!), but you can still incorporate them into your life, and you'll know intuitively whether or not you're accomplishing them, because your joy will increase. What are your desires? List them out!

Action-oriented: Your goals should also be action-based. In other words, they should be something you have to do—hands on. In our examples so far, you have to actually exercise, eat and keep track of how many fruits and vegetables you've eaten, and measure out the food.

There will be times, though, especially when you're just beginning work on a new change or having trouble making a change in an area, when you may want to set more of a cognitive goal—you know, food for thought, get that brain working. For

> There are also some really cool tools available for measuring food portions—plates and bowls that mark serving sizes for common foods right on the dish. One such creation is the Diet Plate. Bad name. Good tool.

instance, if you're having trouble meeting your goals and don't know why, figure it out! Stop and think about why you're not meeting them, and what you can do to start making these changes. This is the cognitive part of this—figuring out why you're not moving forward, and coming up with a plan that will work for you. Sometimes cognitive work will also entail doing some research on a topic to help you better understand why or how to make a particular change. For instance, maybe you've got a goal to begin strength training. You know its benefits, but you have no clue what the difference is between your biceps and hamstrings, let alone which exercises to use to strengthen each of them. This is where the cognitive work comes in. Either purchase a good fitness magazine or book, or get on the Internet. Or hire a personal trainer or wellness coach (I know where you can get a really good wellness coach!). Once you've got a better understanding of what you need to do, you can then move forward with more action-oriented goals.

Realistic: Your goals are the bridge that connects the gap of where you are now and where you want to be three months from now. How realistic they are should also be based on this premise. Actually, I include The Three R's in this stage: Realistic, Reasonable, and Reachable. Including The Three R's just reinforces the need to have goals that fit you and fit the three-month time span. While you should stretch and

> "Nine out of 10 of the greatest accomplishments of mankind were done on a deadline."--Bill Phillips

challenge yourself, creating totally unrealistic goals will only set you up for disappointment.

Remember, goals are not written in stone. You may reach a three-month goal in just two months. That's okay! You can either keep that three-month goal for accountability to your new habit as you move into the maintenance phase, or check it off as "done," then create a new goal at a higher level. At the other end of the spectrum, you may find after a month or so, that you over-stretched yourself and made an unreasonable three-month goal. That's okay, too. Revise it to be reachable for you.

Time-oriented: Setting a deadline for your goal is the framework on which it's built. Having a deadline is like having an accountability partner. It keeps you on track for reaching your goals. This is why you set three-month and weekly goals. Three months and one week are your deadlines. Without deadlines, you have nothing to work for.

> There is a constant reassessment process that must go on in this journey.

As a writer, I know this fact very well! If my editors handed out assignments and told us to get them done "whenever," do you think there would be the plethora of magazines lining supermarket racks? Setting a deadline or basing your goals on a timeline is a necessary component to success.

Now what? You've designed your wellness vision and mission; you've set your goals. There's only one thing left to do. Just do it! Here's where the wheels really start moving! You must now grab a hold of that steering wheel and put your plan into action. But this isn't one of those "move forward and never look back" missions. While you're moving ahead, you must also stop for breaks to determine if where you're headed is the right direction for you. There is a constant reassessment process that must happen during this journey. You take a step and you stop and assess. You take a step and you stop and reflect. You take a step and you stop and determine if what you're doing is working. Is it taking you where you want to go? Are you hurdling your obstacles? Or are you still getting stuck in the muddy quagmire of excuses? Is what you're doing moving you closer to meeting your three-month goals? Does it mesh with your purpose and mission? Does it reflect your vision?

A Coaching Moment

During your journey, ask yourself the following questions:
- What excuses am I still hanging onto?
- Am I asking myself powerful questions?
- Are my weekly goals moving me closer to my three-month goals?
- Are my goals reflecting my mission, purpose, and vision?
- Are my goals reasonable, realistic, and reachable?
- Are they SMART goals?

It's important to have a place to organize your goals. If you choose not to get the companion workbook, use a blank journal or notebook. Organize it, personalize it, and make it your own! Another must-have: a planner with a calendar to schedule those "appointments" and work on "de-fluffing" that schedule!

For the Gadget Gal, a Personal Digital Assistant, a.k.a. a PDA, is a great way to plan and organize your goals and time. If you don't already own one, be sure to try as many as possible before making a purchase to make sure it "fits" you.

For the woman who wants or needs more, consider hiring a wellness coach, whose job is to help you define and set your goals—and then reach them!

I hope the meaning of this book has truly come to light by now—if not, I'm not doing a very good job getting my point across! As women, we try to squeeze ourselves into molds that were never intended for us—regardless of what the media or anyone else tries to make us believe. Your journey through life is *your* journey, and should not be

> ## Cool Tools
>
> Whether you're a paper person or a gadget gal (and you know who you are!), having the right tools will help you establish and reach your new goals. There are several products, workbooks, and journals on the market that will help you get going and stick to your journey. Many of them have their own agendas, though, so just make sure they don't contradict what you're trying to accomplish. Of course, I could recommend the corresponding *Squeezing Your Size 14 Self into a Size 6 World Companion* Workbook (that's available at www.championpress.com) but that just wouldn't seem fair. Would it?

based on some cover model (she's got her own journey). While I believe the media has done a good job in confusing us, I also believe they think they're giving us what we want, and that ultimately, it's our responsibility to stop supporting what they're selling if we feel it's unhealthy for us.

Hopefully you're experiencing one of those "A-Ha!" moments during our time together, where you realize that you do in fact hold the key to your journey. With God as your co-pilot, you can and will be the woman He intends for you to be.

Stepping Stones

- Create your Wellness Vision.
- Determine your personal mission and purpose.
- Design your goals and action plan.
- Continue to ask yourself powerful questions.
- Just do it!

PART FOUR

Food, Fitness & You

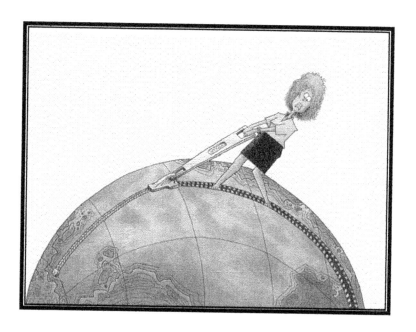

CHAPTER TWELVE
Never Say Die-t

Have you ever noticed what the first three letters of "diet" spell? And isn't that appropriate? Each time we diet, it chips away at our spirits, bit by bit, causing a slow death.

There are many reasons for this. For starters...who actually *enjoys* dieting? Recently, we were at a local ice cream parlor and I overheard a woman say she was all "psyched up" to start a new diet (then she made mention of one of those shakes...and I don't mean an ice cream shake). That's exactly what we have to do—psych ourselves up for it. It's like standing on the dock over a crisp, clear lake. We know it's going to be frigid, but we hope the pay-off—cooling our bodies or getting some exercise—is worth the price. So we stand there trying to talk ourselves into taking the plunge. We take a few deep breaths, rub our bodies down, take another deep breath, close our eyes, and...jump! That's how most of us approach dieting. We contemplate it for a few days (or weeks). We set "the date," and mark it on our calendars. We eat everything and anything—all our favorite foods and even our not-so-favorite foods—prior to "the date," because they're gone forever once "the date" arrives. We talk ourselves into it by saying, "It's only food." We consider the ads and how they show the delicious-looking bars and shakes—just like candy bars and milk shakes—only we can lose weight snarfing down these confections. We'll feel like we're cheating, but we won't really be. It's "the diet."

A Coaching Moment
How do you psych yourself up to begin a diet?

Let's take a moment to play out this dieting scene, starring…you! As "the date" approaches, you start to feel a little bit of anxiety. The family reunion is next week and you know your aunt's famous pies will be there—not to mention Uncle Joe's finger-lickin' bar-b-q chicken. Can you resist? Maybe you should reset "the date." Nope. If you don't do it now, you never will. There will always be some excuse. So when the big morning arrives, you take a few deep breaths, rub your body down, take another deep breath, close your eyes, and…you whip that baby up and take your first big gulp. *Mmm…hmmm. It's kind of chalky,* you think. *Sort of sticks to the roof of my mouth. Kind of has a bad after taste. Well, it'll be worth it if it works.*

For your mid-morning snack, at which time you're absolutely starving (those shakes really aren't so filling), you rip open the wrapper on one of the bars. *Hmm. Looks pretty good,* you think. *They do look bigger on TV, though.* You take a bite. You decide it's better than the shake, with just a *slightly* chalky texture (we won't mention the after-taste).

Thus goes your first day, alternating bars with shakes, until your optional evening meal, at which time you freak out. I mean, can you really trust yourself with *real food*? But wow! Are you ever hungry. The problem is, the family wants pizza, which isn't "allowed" for you. However, you convince yourself you can handle the scintillating scent of your favorite toppings, melted cheese, crispy crust, and spicy sauce wafting through the house while you choke down a naked, broiled chicken breast and steamed veggies.

The pizza arrives and you've got a knot in your stomach— partly from anxiety over wanting a slice, but knowing you couldn't live with the guilt and feelings of failure, and partly from being truly hungry. You somehow manage to jump that hurdle and you feel proud to have made it through your first day.

Three days later...

You've tried every flavor bar and shake and decide you like the chocolate ones best (of course!). So you buy all chocolate flavored supplements for the next week. So far so good—and not one "cheating moment."

One week later...

You never want to see another chocolate *anything* again!

Family Reunion weekend...

You come armed with your supplies—plenty of bars and shakes to get you through the day. *Mmm-Mmm. All that food looks so good!* You decide to have your evening meal at noon instead, and begin loading up your plate. You then begin to wonder why in the world you ever told everyone that you were on this marvelous new diet. You feel as though all eyes are on you, watching what you're taking.

You make it through lunch, and then dessert is unveiled. *Dessert and diet certainly don't seem to mesh,* you think. *And everyone stared enough through lunch. Maybe I could just wait until everyone has taken their dessert then nonchalantly saunter on over, sneak a piece of pie, and hide it on my way to the bathroom.* After considering this option for a moment, you slap yourself in disgust. *So this is what it's come to—sneaking food and eating in the bathroom?* You choose to forego reputation and stand back, waiting until everyone else is eating their dessert so they're less likely to focus on what you're doing.

The rest of the afternoon doesn't go much better. Snacks are left out for party-goers to munch on. That's not a problem though. You ate enough to feed the United States Army, Navy, Marines, Air Force, and—heck, why not throw in the Coast Guard—at noontime (and since you couldn't decide between the cake and pie, you ended up sneaking off with a slice of each, and shamefully shoving them down your throat while you sat in a toilet stall—feet up on the toilet so no one could tell you were in there—unless, of course, they overheard the grunting), and you've been extremely uncomfortable since. You're invited to join your cousins in the pool. *Me? Get into a bathing suit? First of all, I haven't lost enough weight yet. Second of all, I look as though I'm six months pregnant with all the food sitting in my stomach.* So instead, you sit there, hoping someone will come and talk with you. Occasionally someone will stop and say hello, ask how you're doing—you know, "weather" talk.

As the afternoon wears on, everyone is encouraged to fill their plates again before heading home. *Should I? I mean, a little while ago I could barely move, I ate so much. But now, well, I do feel as though I could eat a little something. I should just have a shake or bar, though. I really should not eat any more real food. But I've already blown it for today. Ah. Why not?* So you load up again, joking to everyone how you may as well *really* blow your diet today—you'll make up for it tomorrow.

The next day...

Upon awaking, you feel sick and bloated. It's a "fat day." According to the mirror, you don't look any different, but the mirror lies. You know you're fatter. All that food you ate yesterday is just sticking to your hips and waist like Velcro®. You deserve this, however. It's part of your punishment. Although you're hungry, you decide you're not even worth a diet shake and you skip breakfast. By mid-morning you're *really* hungry, so you allow yourself half a bar. At noon you drink half a shake and dump the rest so you don't drink anymore of it (you can't be trusted, you know). But the other half of that bar is staring at you, so you eat it to get it over with and so you don't have to worry about it. You spend the afternoon running errands and out of the house so you don't have to think about food. You subsist on coffee and gum for the rest of the day.

One month later...

You've dropped a few pounds and you know you could lose more if you stick with it, but the old shake and bar routine is getting old. Chalk it up to lack of willpower or a lack of interest. Whichever it is, it's just yet another notch on the bedpost of failure. You return to your old eating habits, which immediately include an entire pint of Ben and Jerry's New York Super Fudge Chunk® due to feelings of depression and self-pity, and within two months you will have regained all the lost weight and then some.

Do you recognize yourself in our dieting scenario at all? A little bit? A lot? Chances are, most of us can relate to something there. Let's take a moment and analyze this whole dieting scene. Let's break it apart, comb through it, and see exactly…

Why Diets Don't Work

Diets set us up for failure. By eliminating major foods or food groups—many times ones that in their natural state, are very healthy—human nature, will cause us to want those foods even more. This causes anxiety and stress, which in turn feed into (no pun intended!) emotional eating. And so the cycle starts all over again. The whole family-reunion day is a good example of this. When presented with all that "forbidden" food, you crumbled. Had you not been depriving yourself, you could have made a rational decision to take only what and how much you really wanted and knew would satisfy you. When you don't own a list of "forbidden" foods, you don't have to feel guilty about having dessert or a hot dog on a special occasion. When you diet and "cheat," you fail, thus becoming a "failure," perpetuating the whole cycle of diet-lose-gain-fail. Food should not be an area where we're graded on a pass/fail basis.

Diets are boring. By the end of our dieting scene, you were getting tired of eating the same thing day in and day out. And who wouldn't? By restricting the foods you're eating, you limit what is "allowed." So whether it's bars and shakes, mostly protein, mostly high fat, or mostly grapefruit, it eventually gets…yawn…boring…which brings me to the next point…

Diets don't make sense. Does it make sense to eat so much food high in saturated fat, for instance, when we know the havoc it wreaks on the body? Despite claims that dieters' cholesterol and triglyceride levels are okay (and even go down), a good long-term study still remains among the missing (although, at the time of this writing, is just beginning— finally!). And let's not even mention what eating all that fat does to our intestines (gurgle, gurgle). This is just one example. If a diet is leaving out major foods or food groups, especially ones that are known to be healthy (Run! It's an apple!), cue in to your common sense and ask does this diet make sense?

A Coaching Moment

Before getting drawn into the latest dieting scheme, ask yourself, "Does this make sense?" Rather than allowing your emotions to drag you into it, use your common sense and think about it. Does it eliminate or severely restrict healthy foods or food groups? Does it match your personality? Does it require you to do things, such as count calories, that you know won't work for you? Does it give you options? Does it make too-good-to-be-true promises? Consider journaling all this out. Seeing it on paper can be a good reality check!

Diets are stressful. Anyone who has been on a diet, or who has lived with someone on a diet, knows what I mean. It's comparable to someone who is trying to quit smoking. We're trying to take away (because that's what diets do—they take away), something very valuable to us. What makes it even worse is we have to eat to live. We have to go into the grocery store, with their very heavily marketed schemes. We have to prepare meals. We have to get together with family and friends.

So much in our society centers around food. I don't necessarily think this is a bad thing. Food is a part of our celebrations. We shouldn't fear food. But we also need to get out of the "all-you-can-eat" mode.

Diets are not satisfying. This goes along with the boring point. If the diet is boring, we're not being satisfied. We have so much low fat and no fat food available to us these days, and we're eating so much of it, but we're still not satisfied. Experts feel there are two reasons why, even with all the low fat foods currently available, obesity is still on the rise. One is that we think that if it's low or no fat, we can eat more of it. Consequently, we eat as many calories as we did before. The other reason is that we're not being satisfied. Fat helps fill us up. So much low and no fat doesn't give us that feeling of being satisfied. After so long of not feeling satisfied, what do we do? Dare I say it? The "B" word...binge!

Have you ever read the fine print on most diet ads? While the once-fat-now-thin spokesperson flits around on your TV screen, telling you how great the product is and how her life has changed forever, the words, "Results not typical" faintly appear, hoping you won't notice. Why do you put yourself through that type of torture, when the companies themselves are telling you that chances are, you will not succeed?

Diets make you want to cheat. This goes along with the satisfaction thing. If you're not being satisfied, eventually, you're going to look for a way to become satisfied. And because diets don't allow certain foods, the dissatisfaction comes from not getting a variety of foods, as well as not feeling full. Which, again, leads to that "B" word.

Diets are all about head games. Or maybe I should say they play off your emotions, since, when it comes to diets, not too many of us even use our heads! It begins with the commercial, the ad, the display in the store. "I lost 150 pounds and 987 inches in a month," the buff, bikini clad bombshell claims in the photo, "by drinking three shakes and popping 15 pills a day." Okay, remember my "diets don't make sense" point? How many people do you know who lost a lot of weight really fast and kept it off? And does it make sense to only drink shakes (or whatever!) or pop pills to be thin? Diet marketers hope to hook you in the core of your emotions. And they're doing a good job of it. We spend $30-$60 billion a year on diet aids! They get us where it hurts the most, and lure us into their trap…time after time after time. Not to mention they're getting rich, while we get nowhere in our quest for wellness. In fact, we may very well endanger our health!

Diets don't teach you about life-long eating. How many of us could live on chalky shakes and bars, broth, or grease-laden garbage indefinitely? No! We go on the diet, because we know it's short-term. There will be an end to it. And that's exactly why they don't work. They are short-term, and they don't teach us anything about real life eating.

Diets are about the quick-fix. While we say we want to keep the weight off, we keep gravitating to the "magic bullet" type diets. Ones that promise quick weight loss. Research has shown time and again that a safe—and more lasting—weight loss is one to two pounds a week. People who are making healthier choices and putting their wellness plans into place—and into action—are the ones who tend to be the most successful. It's about changing your entire life—not about restricting what goes into your mouth.

Diets are deceptive. Many of us like diets, because they offer a security blanket—in a sort of twisted way. This blanket is soft and fuzzy on the outside, but cold and scratchy on the inside. Having a diet plan gives a feeling of security, knowing that you don't have to go through this on your own. You've got your guide telling you exactly what you need to do, and that's comforting. But it doesn't take long to realize that you *are* on your own! You are the one having to put the plan into action, a plan, that after all, doesn't really fit you. Which brings me to our next point…

> No one else's plan will fit you as well as the plan you put together for yourself!

Diets are just another example of trying to squeeze into someone else's mold. There are diets that claim to be right for everyone. Then there are those that claim to fit *you* based on some questionnaire you've filled out. But with all the thousands of dynamics associated with life and eating, how can any plan that someone else has created truly fit you? Yes, some come very close—close enough to even help a little. But no one else's plan will fit you as well as the plan you put together for yourself!

Stepping Stones

- Diets set us up for failure.
- Diets are boring.
- Diets don't make sense.
- Diets are stressful.
- Diets are not satisfying.
- Diets make you want to cheat.
- Diets are all about head games.
- Diets don't teach you about lifelong eating.
- Diets are all about the quick-fix.
- Diets are deceptive.
- Diets are just another example of trying to squeeze into someone else's mold.

CHAPTER THIRTEEN

What's Your Eating Personality?

As I said in the previous chapter, I believe one reason women tend to be drawn to diets is that it gives them some sort of security—structure in an otherwise unstructured, hectic, chaotic world. It clearly lays out what is allowed and what's not. And for those of us who feel out-of-control around food, this is a welcome thing. But as we've all attested to, we quickly begin to see that while it appears at first that such tight structure works, the walls eventually begin to slowly crumble away, until we finally are back at square one—except that we feel even worse about ourselves than we did before we started the diet.

Each of us has a unique style of eating. No, I'm not talking about whether or not you talk with your mouth full, or whether you sip instead of slurp. I'm talking about your eating patterns throughout the day. In my coaching experience, I've been able to pinpoint a number of varieties of eating personalities or styles (some healthy, some not-so-healthy), including the grazer, the three-squares-a-day, the three-squares-a-day-plus-snacks, the eat-only-when-I'm-hungry, the skipper, the grab-n-go, and the don't-eat-till-I'm-practically-dead.

You may or may not be one of these types. You may exhibit traits from two or more—multiple personalities! As you read through these personalities and styles, think about your current eating habits, and how they help or hinder your Wellness Vision.

The Grazer

Think "cow" here. I don't mean the grazer is a cow—I mean she eats like one. If you're a grazer, you tend to pick at things all day long, without really eating what anyone would call a "real meal." The world is your pasture, and you're there to graze upon it. This works for some people. Scientifically, one could say that this personality keeps her metabolism revved up, providing a constant, steady supply of fuel. However, for those who aren't natural grazers and have a problem with portion control, or if you tend to eat subconsciously (we'll talk more about this phenomenon in a moment), this probably isn't the best eating pattern. Many of us have been conditioned to eat meals, so when we attempt a trial at grazing, we're hit with the hard realization that come day's end, we've actually consumed ten complete meals. Nope. Grazing isn't for everyone. If you try grazing, and feel out-of-control with it, stop. Find a personality that fits you.

The Three-Squares-a-Day

Three square meals a day is what many, if not most, of us were raised on. Somewhere along the line, either while we were kids, or in some magazine touting the latest dieting tricks, snacking become evil. Snacks became what was making us fat. I recently read an article where a woman, who had gastric bypass surgery (you know, where they chop your stomach down to thumb-size?), offered tips to readers. In a nutshell, her advice was, "Do not snack!" Perhaps this is what worked for her. Maybe due to her situation (the surgery), this is what she had to do. But for someone to give advice specific to her situation, and apply it to the general population is wrong. Most experts will tell you that snacking is fine, beneficial even. It's what you're eating for snacks on a regular basis that can cause problems. If you tend to be a three-squares kinda gal, ask yourself if it's working for you. Do you get hungry between meals? Do you feel your energy wane between meals? Are you so hungry by the next meal that you tend to grab whatever is available or totally go off the deep end and binge? If so, consider changing personalities to the next one…

Three-Squares-a-Day-Plus-Snacks
(a.k.a. five to six small meals a day)

This is currently popular among the health and fitness field. It can also be interpreted as the "five to six small meals a day" personality. Why do we love this one? Perhaps because it allows us to eat, without feeling deprived, but we still keep a bit of tradition in there. Health and fitness experts like to promote this idea, because research has shown that eating often, can help keep your metabolism revved up. And not just your metabolism, but your energy and brain power, as well. The key, however, is to make healthy choices most of the time. Grabbing donuts and Hershey Kisses® at the office each day doesn't make ideal fuel for your engine. You want that engine to purrrrrr…so feed it well. One catch—the size of the meals and snacks counts. Notice it says five to six *small* meals. So if your typical meal more closely resembles a Thanksgiving spread, you'll need to re-evaluate the amount of food you're eating at each sitting.

Eat-Only-When-I'm-Hungry

This one makes sense: fill your belly when you're hungry. That's what God created that little uncomfortable feeling in the depths of our gut for. Right? Right. But the problem is that due to our crazy beliefs about our bodies and what we should and shouldn't be eating, and our past attempts to squelch any feeling of hunger we possess, many of us have desensitized our hunger cues. Whether it's because we've learned to ignore it, or whether we just constantly eat whatever, whenever, we have a difficult time picking up on our bodies' natural cues. We've lost our natural body wisdom. I personally recommend that no matter what personality you are, you can learn to re-distinguish and re-connect with your feeling of hunger.

The Skipper

While the name implies the skipper is head of her ship, this skipper is anything but. The skipper tends to skip at least breakfast, grabbing whatever monster-sized caffeine-infused, sugar-loaded beverage is available at the time. She may eat lunch—if she doesn't have a meeting or deadline she's behind on. And dinner is whatever—usually the drive-through, order-in pizza, or something left-over off her kids' plates. The skipper usually claims that her schedule is just too busy to allow time to eat. She can be confused with the "Grab-n-Go" personality, and the two often overlap with each other.

Grab-n-Go

Many of today's food manufacturers cater to the grab-n-go style person. From grab-n-go yogurts to grab-n-go breakfast bars, a girl could easily live on prepackaged-straight-from-the-box food. The problem, however, is just that—most of what she's grabbing is prepackaged, which means it's not fresh and usually includes a bunch of extra garbage—artificial colors, preservatives, and loads of sugar and salt...albeit vitamin fortified. And as the old saying goes, "You are what you eat." If you fill up on prepackaged foods, you miss out on many essential micronutrients and fiber that are found naturally in whole foods, such as fruits, veggies, and whole grains. And enough studies have been done so that we can confidently say that an eating plan that includes lots of these natural and whole foods decreases one's risk of disease.

Don't-Eat-Till-I'm-Practically-Dead

This person puts off eating, much like the skipper does, but even more so. While she claims it's because of her overloaded schedule, the deeper issue is trying to avoid food, in an attempt to control her weight. But as we all know, the most likely end result is...the "B" word. After succeeding at being a meal-time ice princess and preventing a utensil from passing her lips, the don't-eat-till-I'm-practically-dead type loses it and eats whatever is lurking inside the refrigerator, freezer, pantry, cupboards, and any hide-it-from-the-kids-and-hubby nooks and crannies. Hence, she ends up eating as many calories—or more—at one sitting as she would have had she eaten regularly throughout the day. And chances are, there aren't too many fruits, vegetables, or whole grains that find their way into her binge fest, either.

A Coaching Moment

What's your eating personality? Maybe it's a combination of two or more of the styles mentioned. Maybe it's a totally different, all-your-own style. Think about what personality most naturally fits you—and what style you've been trying to squeeze yourself into. If you feel as though you've been following your natural personality, what are some steps you can take to bring your style more in line with your wellness goals?

How to Use Your Personality to Your Advantage

Do you recognize yourself in any of these eating personalities or styles? Is there one that particularly stands out? Is the outstanding one your natural style? Or is it the one you've been trying to squeeze yourself into? While there is no one perfect personality, do you see which ones have more potential to support healthy habits?

You may discover that your *current* style of eating isn't what really comes *naturally* to you. You may be forcing your eating style into a mold based on your schedule, for instance. Maybe you've been living as a grab-n-goer or skipper, but know that you perform best as a grazer. But because grazing doesn't work with your work schedule, you just don't eat until you get home at night. This all goes back to having a plan and doing a little critical thinking to find ways to instill healthier habits. For instance, if grazing doesn't mesh with your schedule, consider the next closest thing—either five to six small meals a day or the three squares plus snacks. These two styles offer a more defined pattern of eating, often meshing better with a typical work environment.

On the flip side, perhaps you'll find what comes *naturally* to you, isn't what is *best* for you. This all comes back to that balance thing. There are many things in our lives that come naturally, that aren't necessarily healthy. Much of this is simply a matter of conditioning over time and establishing certain habits. The key is to find what fits you, your schedule, and your wellness goals and desires.

A Coaching Moment

Is your schedule preventing you from establishing healthy eating habits? How can you create a more wellness-conducive work environment for yourself—one that will allow you the opportunity to feed your body what it needs to perform at its best?

Part of the problem with many diets and pre-made eating programs is that they don't take the individual into account. They limit your choices of food. They tell you what, how much, and when to eat. At just a smidgen under 5'4" with a medium frame size, I certainly don't need as many calories as a woman who is 5'8" with a large frame size. And while my personality may prefer three squares plus three snacks (yes, I snack at night if I'm hungry—healthy snacking, but snacking none the less), the other woman may prefer to graze all day, but not eat past 7 PM. And each style works for each of us—even my night snacking, which has been long hailed as a contributor of being over weight. And yes, if I was snarfing down a pint of Ben and Jerry's® every night, this would cause problems. Instead, when I feel hungry, I eat something light—fruit, a small handful of nuts or a string cheese—just enough to take off the edge, especially if I'm not going to bed right away. This is what works for me. You need to find what works for you.

A Coaching Moment

Think back to a time in your life when you were happiest with your body. Jog your memory—what nutritional habits did you have at that time? Were they healthy? What can you draw from this past experience and how can you apply it to what you want to accomplish today? Plan out how you can start applying these changes today.

Stepping Stones

- We each have a unique way of eating and relating to food.
- We often eat "subconsciously," not really thinking about what we're eating.

CHAPTER FOURTEEN

Create Your Own Personalized, Real-Life Eating Plan

L et's face it. Not everything in this book will apply to you, nor will everything be entirely helpful. But hopefully I'm giving you some tools to put into your own personal toolbox. These tools work well for tailoring your eating personality and style, furthering your journey to wellness. Rather than throwing out or tossing aside what you feel doesn't fit you at the moment, I suggest tucking it away into a special compartment in your toolbox. Remember, you're changing. What fits and works for you now, may not further along on your journey—and visa versa.

Trust yourself. This is a biggie. Diets scream at us, "Hey! You can't trust yourself to eat what you're supposed to (because if you could, you wouldn't be where you are now), so let us show you how (hee, hee, hee…)." And while they're saying this, they're thinking, "Suckers. We'll just lure them into this new diet, then when they fail, have something else to hook them with."

In order to move ahead, you must *trust yourself!* Forget about what other people, ads, and articles say. Don't let past "failures" color your identity—at least not in a bad way. Take those experiences and use them to create new successes. You *can* trust yourself with an empty house and a full fridge. You *can* trust yourself at your cousin's wedding smorgasbord. You *can* trust yourself with the barbecue at your family reunion, with the all-you-can-eat buffet at your favorite restaurant, and with your church potluck. Part of the problem has been that you've *allowed* yourself to believe that you *couldn't* be trusted. You've told yourself that food has some magical, undeniable power over you.

> You *can* trust yourself with an empty house and a full fridge. You *can* trust yourself at your cousin's wedding smorgasbord. You *can* trust yourself with the barbecue at your family reunion, with the all-you-can-eat buffet at your favorite restaurant, and with your church potluck.

You've come to believe that you aren't to be trusted around food, that you can't control yourself. Oh, maybe you can control yourself temporarily, but just you wait until you get yourself alone with that cheesecake. Watch out!

A Coaching Moment

Get your journal and write out what you feel like when you're around food. Do you feel out-of-control? Do you feel comforted by food? Do you have a love-hate relationship with food? Do you fear food? In what roots do you think these feelings lie? Sometimes, the way we see food today has a lot to do with how we saw food as a child. Did you grow up in a large family and the motto was "Get it now or get nothing?" Were your parents really strict about what you ate or when you ate? Was food used as a reward and/or punishment? These early experiences with food can carry over into adulthood. See if you can relate any childhood memories to your current relationship with food. Take a realistic, thoughtful look at your life now. How can you change your mindset about food?

Pay attention to what your body is telling you. Learn to pick up on hunger cues. In return, responding to them will help put eating back into its proper perspective. It will become more satisfying as you realize that you're meeting a need, not just fulfilling a self-motivated indulgence. But as I mentioned before, many of us couldn't recognize true hunger if it hit us over the head and shouted, "Here I am! Feed me!" If you've been suppressing your feelings of hunger, it's time for you to increase your self-awareness. Place your hand over your tummy, and concentrate on that part of your body. How does it feel? I don't mean what does your hand feel...I mean, what does that entire part of your body feel like inside? Take a deep breath. Is your stomach talking? Do you hear rumbling? Squeaking? Gurgling? Does it feel uncomfortable? Is it more like a gassy feeling, or a "feed me" feeling? When was the last time you ate? If you just ate an hour ago, is it reasonable that you could be hungry again? What did you eat? Did you have something "fluffy"—no substance to it (hey—"fluff" can apply to food, too!)? Was it something high in sugar so that it gave you a

> Larger value sizes and bulk sizes are not always your best bargain. While they may be a monetary deal (and even then, you need to check the unit price), they're not always a very good health deal. If you find that having the extra large quantity under your roof just provides more temptation than it's worth, then don't give in to the financial savings you get at the store.

good sugar buzz, but then quickly left you lagging? Learn to recognize the "feed me" feeling, and distinguish it from normal digestion. If you find that you just can't seem to identify your true hunger pangs, seek help from a qualified dietician, physician, or therapist.

> Simple, refined carbohydrates and sugars tend to pass quickly through us, hence, causing the spike in blood sugar, a.k.a., the sugar high, buzz, boost...and the sudden, plummeting downfall. Notice I said refined carbohydrates. Those are the white flour products. Whole grains are a different—and much healthier—story. Whole grains contain the bran and germ of the grain, which contain not only fiber, but also lots of vitamins, minerals, and micronutrients that not even the "enriched" white products can imitate. Try easing into using whole grain products by mixing half whole grain with half the white counterpart. Pasta, rice, or cereals are all good things to start with.

Follow your instincts. Some would argue that as humans, we don't have instincts. But I think no matter what you call it, we all have some degree of self-wisdom. In the process of losing trust in ourselves, however, we've also lost this wisdom. Following your instincts involves learning to trust yourself, learning to listen to your body, and learning to listen to your intuition. Intuitive eating, applies these aspects by cueing you on when, what, and how much to eat. But you have to be conscious (see below) of what you're doing, and not just flitting through your day unaware. This all goes back to planning and de-cluttering your schedule. See how it's all inter-related?

Eat with consciousness. Quick! Tell me what you ate last night for supper. Waaaaiiiiting…can't seem to remember? What about lunch? Breakfast? Snacks? If you have to stop and really think—and especially if you can't remember at all— about what you ate less than 24 hours ago, chances are you're eating subconsciously. All this means is that you're not thinking about what you're putting into your mouth. You're

---

Looking at Labels

Manufacturers and advertisers can often be "slight of hand" artists, tricking us into thinking what we're buying is healthy. For instance, if you pack juice boxes, make sure what you're packing really is juice. If it says "drink" or "cocktail" anywhere on the label, it isn't all juice, and is in fact, mostly sugar water and artificial flavoring. "One hundred percent juice" must be stamped on the package to count as a serving of fruit. Another one is "wheat" bread. If the bread is dark, and we see "wheat" on the front of the packaging, we assume it's healthy. Wrong! Any bread made with wheat is wheat bread. It must say "100% Whole Wheat" to be the healthier version. If it doesn't, it's just refined, white flour that's been colored with a caramel coloring or molasses to make it dark. Here's another one: "all natural." Sugar is "all natural," but I'll bet you didn't think that's what they were talking about when they stamped that on the label! The term "all natural" simply means that the product doesn't have any artificial flavors, colors or preservatives. Become a label reader. The first few ingredients will tell you what the product is really made of since ingredients are listed in order by the amount the product contains.

---

grabbing whatever is available and convenient or looks good at the time. Tell me this—what's for supper tonight? Tomorrow night? Planning what you'll eat ahead of time leaves less chance of shoving any old thing into your mouth when the mood strikes. This also gives you a higher guarantee that you'll be planning healthier, more nutrient-packed meals and snacks. *But I don't have time to plan ahead like that!* If you're still using *that* old excuse, go back and read the first section of this book! I've said it before, and I'll say it again: taking the time to plan saves time in the long run. Try it!

Add color to your plan. If you're all set with the amount of food, but want to increase the quality of what you're putting in your mouth, try eating according to the rainbow. By consciously including a variety of *naturally* colored (FD&C Yellow #5 & #6 don't count!) foods—red, orange, yellow, blue, green, and purple—you'll automatically go for the fruits and vegetables, upping your nutrient and fiber intake. By the way, this is a great way to get kids to eat their fruits and veggies, too! Take them to the local farmer's market and see how many different colored produce you can find.

A Coaching Moment

Before you set sail on your next diet, ask yourself:

- Is this a quick fix?
- Will this instill lifetime changes?
- Does this diet make sense?
- Does it cut out food or food groups that are normally considered healthy?
- Does it drastically cut calories?
- Does it make promises of quick, permanent weight loss?
- Does it fit my personality?
- Does it encourage healthy, moderate activity?
- Does it require pills, powders, or commercialized, prepackaged food?

If you answered yes to any of these questions, take a second look and reconsider your choice.

Don't think of foods in terms of good or bad. All our lives we've made distinctions between good food and bad food. French fries—bad, apples—good (well, depending on what diet plan you're following!), hot fudge sundaes—bad, broccoli—good. The problem with sorting food into "good" and "bad" categories is that when you choose something from the "bad" column, it reflects onto you, and you are now "bad." Then you have to deal with that guilt issue. You feel like you're a failure, you're never going to succeed or measure up…same old story, new time and place. By eliminating forbidden foods from your mindset, you now free yourself to eat a wide variety of food—whether it's healthy or not. The key, however, is moderation and balance (you knew there had to be a catch, huh?). Try to eat well—meaning healthy, nutrient-packed foods—most of the time. Now, "most of the time" can be rather subjective, since technically, 51 percent is a majority. But most experts agree that "most" in this case is around 80-90 percent of the time. Some people choose one day during the week where they allow themselves to eat all their special treats. Others eat a little special treat everyday. Others just make it a habit to eat healthy, but don't panic if their normally healthy option isn't available. It can take time to stop dividing food into "good" and "bad," but as you'll see, it opens up so many more options—and removes the guilt!

Calories In/Calories Out. While many diets try to disprove this claim, to my knowledge, so far, none have been able to do so. And while we may find this is not true someday (due to more in-depth research), at this time, I can tell you that ultimately, when it comes to weight loss, the basic premise is calories in/calories out. If you're eating fewer calories than you put out (or the other way around: you put out more calories than you're putting in), chances are, you're going to lose weight. What kind of weight you're losing will depend on how many calories you're taking in and whether or not you're exercising—too few calories and/or no exercise (especially strength training) and you're going to lose some fat, and a lot of water and muscle.

"Quick" weight loss programs depend on this water and muscle loss for their claims, since the body rids itself of these components faster than it does fat. And yes, you can be skinny but fat—you may look thin, but if the weight loss results in a lot of muscle loss, your ratio of fat to lean body tissue will not be desirable. Remember, too, that the quality of your calories is as important as the quantity of them. Quality calories come mostly from whole foods, such as fruits, veggies, whole grains, nuts, legumes, and lean meats and dairy. You can rack up the same number of calories by eating processed, prepackaged foods, but health-wise, they don't come close!

Don't use food—or a lack of it—as punishment. *Today we fast, for yesterday we binged.* Is that your motto for life? Maybe it's an unspoken one. In any case, we tend to punish ourselves when we feel we've either eaten too much, or what we feel is too much of the wrong thing. This happens when we define food as being either "good" or "bad." Or maybe you've just woken up and decided it's a "fat day," so it's time to start that diet, which begins with eating…nothing. I mean, eating makes you fat, so that must be the crux of the problem. Actually, though, studies show that the major root of our problems seems to be lack of physical activity. In fact, did you know you have a higher chance of dying from being skinny and sedentary than you do from being overweight and active? It's true! While being obese and *in*active is one of the top killers, by adding regular, consistent exercise, you can greatly decrease this risk—even surpassing the skinny couch potatoes! In the meantime, stop withholding food in order to punish yourself for overeating or eating a forbidden food or whatever. So you

> Did you know you have a higher chance of dying from being skinny and sedentary than you do from being overweight and active? It's true!

binged. Admit it and move on. And the next time you feel true hunger, eat something healthy—because you're worth it!

A Coaching Moment

When you have a setback, such as cleaning out the frozen food section at your local supermarket, journal out what you were feeling at the time. Were you bored? Depressed? Angry? What *could* you have done instead of raiding the refrigerator (and the pantry, and the cupboards, and the freezer...oh yeah, and under the mattress...)? What *will* you do the next time you feel that way? What did you learn from this setback? Create a plan and use it the next time you find yourself heading for a fridge fest.

Realize that food has no magical power over you. Do you ever feel a sort of magnetic draw to certain foods? Like they're pulling you toward them, leaving you no choice but to eat them? *I have to have seconds and thirds, because I just can't help it.* It's "addicting." While I don't believe in forbidden foods, there is also a flip side (as with everything else), and that is that we can't just eat mounds of anything and everything! This is

> There is a fine line between healthy freedom and unhealthy overindulgence.

where the moderation, a.k.a. balance, comes in. Don't deprive yourself. Got a craving for ice cream? Go for it! But don't use that as an excuse to eat the whole pint (or half gallon), either. Find the balance that works for you. And remember, *you* have the power over food…not the other way around!

Beware of The Nonfat Fad. Low fat and nonfat foods became the trend in health and fitness well over a decade ago. Cookbooks were released touting the low- and nonfat diets' benefits (recipes included), everyone from physicians and dieticians to fitness professionals and health gurus promoted nonfat living. Food manufacturers didn't miss the bandwagon, either, putting out a plethora of low-fat and no-fat options, still available today. Since that time, we seem to have come full-circle. While most of us still agree that we should limit "bad" fats—saturated fats, found in most animal products (meat, eggs, milk, butter), as well as palm and coconut oils, and trans fats, found in anything with hydrogenated oils, such as margarine, nondairy whipped cream, some cereals, and processed foods like cookies, crackers, and pastries—"good" fats are finally getting the credit they deserve—and for good reason.

The no-fat trend seems to have been a bust. With all the available lower-fat options, we have still grown bigger and bigger, smashing even previous obesity records when these options weren't available. There are many reasons for this (including our sit-on-our-butts-all-day society), but one of the biggest is that we seem to think because something is nonfat, it doesn't have calories—and it must be good for us—so we eat more than we would have of the higher fat version. But read the side panel: many lower-fat foods have nearly as many calories as their higher-fat buddies. This is because when they remove the fat, they remove flavor and to make up for lost taste, they load on the sugar and salt.

Fat is also filling to our stomachs, as well as satisfying to our taste buds. Because of the decreased fat and increased sugar, these products tend to go through us faster, making us hungrier, sooner. If you prefer the lower-fat versions, find out what a serving size is and try to stick to it. Ditto on the regular version. You may also want to consider limiting food that comes out of a box, and eat more of the "real thing." Essential fatty acids (EFAs), also known as "good" fats, are essential because our bodies don't produce them—they must come from the foods we eat. They are also essential for optimum health. Their benefits are many, including keeping heart, skin, and immune systems healthy, lowering blood pressure, improving cholesterol, and inhibiting the formation of both leukotrienes, associated with asthma symptoms, and cytokines, associated with cancer.

You can get your "good" fats by eating foods like fish (especially cold-water fish, such as salmon, tuna, mackerel, and sardines); soybeans and soy products; flaxseed and flaxseed oil; soy, corn, safflower, canola, and olive oils; nuts (especially walnuts, almonds, and peanuts), nut butters, and nut oils; avocados; wheat germ; and seeds (sunflower, for instance).

Add to your nutrition plan before you take away from it.
When considering making healthy nutritional changes, it helps many women to add to their plans first, as opposed to taking foods away, which is what diets do. For instance, if you don't normally have a minimum of five servings of fruits and vegetables a day, start adding them until you reach this goal. If you don't currently drink at least eight glasses of water a day, start gradually incorporating them until you've accomplished this goal. What you may find, is that by adding to your nutrition plan first, you end up not eating as much of the less healthy foods, since you are satisfying your hunger and hydration needs with the healthier alternatives.

Think "replace" rather than "eliminate." This is another good tactic, closely related to adding to your plan. Let's take the water goal again. As an example, let's say you currently drink about three glasses of water a day, three cups of coffee, and two sodas. Choose which you want to start cutting back on, coffee or soda. Now let's say you choose soda. For the first week, you replace one of your sodas with a glass of water. By doing this, you'll increase your water intake by a cup, and decrease your soda intake by one. Continue with this type of pattern until you reach your end goal. This is a great way to combine goals and reach more than one at the same time!

Measure if you must. Personally, I would love it if every woman would trust her instincts, and not fret over every little morsel entering her lips. However, we're all as different as we are the same, and some women need to see on paper what they've eaten and their total calories or fat grams. This can be a great motivator for some women, and pave the way for healthy eating. Keeping track of portion sizes and amounts can also be a helpful tool. If you decide to use this method, you must *accurately* measure the food you're eating—and be honest! It will be of no help to write that you ate a cup of pasta, when in fact, it was actually two cups. And record it soon after you eat. It's amazing how we can forget about those broken cookies or the licks off the frosting spatula!

If counting calories isn't your thing, but you feel you need to keep track of the amount you ate, number of servings is another option. You can go by the USDA food pyramid or the Mayo Clinic food pyramid, or others that are available—whichever one you feel most comfortable with. Same advice goes, though, on recording—be honest, and record as you eat. Don't wait until the end of the day. Want another alternative to actually measuring? Try one of the portion plates available on the market. One is called The Diet Plate—bad name, good tool! One catch: you have to actually eat off a plate—not out of a box or pot—to know how much of it you're eating!

Keep a diary. Call it a diary. Call it a journal. Whatever you name it, writing down what you ate, when you ate it, and how you were feeling when you ate it can be a very effective tool. But don't stop there. If you're feeling stressed out, depressed, bored, frustrated, angry, or whatever other emotion we use as an excuse to binge, why not journal out your feelings *before* you hit the fridge? Getting those feelings out on paper can help put things into perspective. It's also a good reminder to put an action plan in place, come up with solutions, and find something other than food to comfort yourself.

A Coaching Moment

If you tend to be an emotional eater, what are some options to binging that you can begin instilling when you feel that draw to hit the kitchen?

Find Non-Food Ways to Reward Yourself...Most of The Time. In many cultures, food is used as a way to celebrate life. Think about our holidays. Most families have certain recipes that are brought out only once or twice a year, for Thanksgiving, Christmas, Hanukkah, Kwanzaa, Easter, Passover...each holiday has its own traditions. We even relate certain foods to other non-holiday celebrations, such as the Super Bowl. Is there anything wrong with this? I don't think so. I believe it's an important part of

> Ultimately, if you've established balanced eating habits, there is no need to reward—or punish—yourself with food—or the lack of it.

our traditions. But when you constantly "reward" yourself with food—usually ending up in an overindulgence of your favorite treats—your life can end up being one big "food fest." Ultimately, this becomes more of a punishment than a reward. Wouldn't it be nice to reward yourself with something you never seem to have time for, like a facial or a massage? How about a new outfit or even something as simple as a bubble bath or coffee with a friend? Try to find alternatives to popping truffles. Now and then, however, getting all gussied up and going out for a nice dinner with your beau, or slowly savoring a slice of your favorite cheesecake *is* just the right reward. It's all about balance!

Allow Yourself To Fall Apart When You Need To. It used to be that men were the only ones who had to hold it all together. Now, however, it seems inappropriate for women to "lose it" now and then. What happens when you hold everything in and transform your emotions into stone? Yep. The old "B" word again! You shove your feelings, being represented by food, further down inside yourself, and in the process, you become more and more unhealthy—both inside and out. If this is you, grab your journal (now!). If you don't have a journal, grab anything that you can write on—a wall, a sheet, your hand, whatever—and write out what has been bothering you since the last time you cried and carried on. Let it *all* out! And cry, baby, cry! Once you've gotten it all out, choose which tools you're going to use the next time you feel like shoving your emotions down your throat. Do you need to talk honestly and frankly with someone about something they're doing (or not doing)? Do you need to make a change in your life? Write down your plan of action and follow through. And when you feel the need to become like stone, don't. Let it out. Begin by journaling or talking to a close friend.

Get Off The Numbers. As women, one of the main issues of our lives is weight. Why is that? When did the almighty scale become so, well, almighty? When did we begin to allow a number to have such power over us? Then there's BMI—Body Mass Index—which is just a height/weight chart. And body composition—a.k.a. body fat. There are lots of numbers we can get hung up on, from these forms of assessment to counting calories and serving sizes to keeping track of reps and sets to measuring our blood pressure, cholesterol, triglycerides, and heart rate. Is it all bad? No! Any of it can be used to healthfully determine if we're on track. And some of it can be lifesaving! But when we become obsessed with numbers and totally depend on them to determine whether or not we're successful on our journey, it becomes unhealthy.

The problem with the scale is that it doesn't differentiate between our weight and height, nor can it tell the difference between our lean tissue—muscle, bones, etc—and fat tissue. Many things also influence our weight from day-to-day, hour-to-hour, including what we've eaten, had to drink, and what stage of the menstrual cycle we're in. If you weight train, the scale will move downward more slowly, because although you're losing fat, you're also adding muscle, and muscle weighs more than fat.

If you tend to get hung up on numbers, find an alternative way to assess your progress. What about your clothes? Are they fitting better—even getting too loose? How about using fitness as your assessment? Can you climb those stairs with ease now, where before, you felt as though you had completed a marathon just carrying a load of wash upstairs? Was the farthest you could walk half a mile when you first started? Now you're jogging two miles!

A Coaching Moment

Are you hung up on numbers? What are some alternative methods you can use to assess your journey's progress? Be creative! It's your journey!

Stepping Stones

- Use the tools that help move you forward in your journey—store the others away for "just in case."
- Pay attention to what your body is telling you.
- Follow your instincts.
- Become an educated consumer.
- Eat with consciousness.
- Don't think of foods in terms of "good" or "bad."
- Don't use food—or a lack of it—as punishment.
- Realize that food has no magical power over you.
- Limit your intake of saturated and trans fats, but be sure to include plenty of the "good" fats—omega-fatty acids and omega-6 fatty acids (both polyunsaturated fats) and monounsaturated fats.
- Try adding to your nutrition plan before you take away from it.
- Think "replace" rather than "eliminate."
- Measure if you must.
- Keep a food diary.
- Find non-food ways to reward yourself.
- Allow yourself to fall apart when you need to…and then pull yourself together and get back on track.
- Try not to rely solely on numbers to tell you whether or not you're health

CHAPTER FIFTEEN

The "Average" Woman's Four-Letter Word

F itness. Exercise. Workout. Is your skin crawling yet? Small beads of sweat starting to form on your brow? Heart racing? What is it about moving our bodies that is so appalling and fearful?

Fitness, I believe, has become the "average" woman's equivalent to a four-letter word. And as a health and fitness professional, I feel the fitness industry is, in large part, to blame. While we've been working hard in our industry to bring fitness to the masses, what we seem to have gotten the best at is making the fit fitter. Today's fitness ideal is so narrow, that only the slimmest, most buff women can even "fit" into it. We've built beautiful gyms, designed awesome equipment for whatever body part it is you want to sculpt, have more personal trainers, group fitness instructors and certifying agencies than ever before, and possess incredible knowledge of exercise and the human body...and yet, we still seem to be missing a huge piece of the puzzle. You!

Personally, I feel a huge part of the problem is the image we've made fitness out to be. Women in skimpy Lycra® outfits, perfectly sculpted everything, big...well, you get the picture. One of the things with making any sort of change, is that the person making the change needs to be able to envision herself in that role. Can you picture yourself being like or looking like the fitness models you see in magazines, videos, or television? Can you envision yourself in that attire, baring all but the bare essentials (I still can't figure out how in the world they dare bounce around, let alone bend over, in some of those outfits!)? One of the reasons I think Richard Simmons has been so popular with women is that, even though he's a man, he's just an "average" kind of guy. And he relates to the "average" person's struggles.

As fitness professionals, we've also gotten really good at the technical aspects of fitness. We can tell you how many reps and sets of what exercise to perform to grow this or that muscle. We can explain the physiology behind fat burning, carbohydrate storage, and ATP production. And we can teach you correct form, posture, and alignment. But we've left out much of the "real-lifeness" that so many people desperately need—sort of like doctors who have bad bedside manners. We've separated fitness from the rest of our lives, making it an entity all to itself, forgetting about the person behind the exercise. By packaging fitness into its own little box, it makes just one more "thing" you should be doing. And if it's not a priority—one of those "must-do-to-live-kind-of-things"—you put it off, saying you'll do it when you've got more time. But as you know, life doesn't seem to let up unless you take over and make it let up.

While I'm on a roll, here's another thing that has bothered me over the years. The fitness industry has become very proficient at pointing the figure at you, telling you to "just make it a priority," and then leave you hanging…not just hanging in the figurative sense, but also hanging your head in shame. We've piled on more guilt, making you feel as though you must be doing something wrong—you're "bad" if you don't workout. And what could possibly be more important than working out, after all? Rather than helping you integrate fitness into your life, we've compounded your guilt for not taking the time to do it, adding to your all ready over-loaded conscience—and schedule. After all, *you* know you *should* be exercising regularly. You know its benefits—how it helps prevent disease, contributes to weight management, and makes you healthier overall. And while you may not know all the ins and outs of every aspect of exercise, chances are, you know how to walk (a very underrated exercise, I might add). Your main problem is probably *when* to fit exercise into your life. *This* we have been remiss on. "Just make it a priority," we say. Yes. It needs to be important to you. You need to *want* to do it and be willing to work on fitting it into your schedule. But fitness doesn't have to match the media's portrayal. And it doesn't have to be an entirely separate entity. It can be woven into your life so that it becomes a natural extension of you.

Lastly (hey, I may as well get it all out!), the fitness industry has also tried to make you, the "average" woman, fit the mold. Rather than try to make fitness fit you, we've tried to squeeze you into a predetermined, "this-is-what-fitness-looks-like" type of box. Obviously, this hasn't worked, since the grand majority of the population does not exercise regularly, if at all. Through my years as a professional, I've had the opportunity to meet many health and fitness professionals (most thanks to the far reach of the internet and email!). I've been pleasantly surprised by many, finding that they've had the same frustrations as I have. But for each positive experience I've witnessed, there has been an equally disappointing one. For instance, there are personal trainers who have told me they would not take on a client who wouldn't complete their "appropriate assessment tests." They likened these assessments to a surgeon's pre-op tests. A surgeon certainly wouldn't perform an operation without baseline assessments, and knowing that it was safe to perform surgery. Right? One of these fitness tests is the body fat measurement. Some trainers feel it to be an absolute, necessary evaluation. If you refused this test, they would not take you on. I feel this is absurd! There are many creative ways, other than just body composition, to evaluate fitness and a client's progress.

Through my research, I've done some informal surveys to try to uncover the pulse of today's women. Guess what one of the tests is that many women hate? You guessed it—body fat measurement! As one woman said to me, "I don't need some stranger pinching my rolls to tell me I'm fat! I know I'm fat—that's why I'm here [to work with a personal trainer]." These women told me that having their body fat done was deflating and de-motivating, and made them want to quit before they even started. Some said it was embarrassing and demeaning to have someone they had just met, get so physically invasive. And they certainly don't appreciate having it done out in the middle of the gym for all the club to see.

On the flip side, body composition can be a motivating factor for other women. While it may be depressing at first to see the actual numbers, they take that initial emotional letdown, and turn it into a fire and determination to meet their goals. The point here is that it should be up to you as to what evaluations and assessments you have done, as long as it is not a medically necessary evaluation (like filling out the health questionnaire). And this is where I feel the personal training aspect of our industry has let you down. As trainers, we have made it all about *our* agenda, rather than listening to you. We create your program around goals *we* set for you, not goals you have created yourself. Rather than looking at possible reasons behind your behaviors (without getting into actual therapy), we tell you what you should be doing differently. Instead of looking at you as a whole person with a whole life, we separate health and fitness from the rest of your life, making no connection the between obstacles at hand and "real life."

How to Choose
A Personal Trainer

If I haven't completely scared you away from looking into hiring a personal trainer, and this is something that interests you, there are a few things to consider when on your hunt. First of all, there are dozens of certifying agencies out there—and more and more join the ranks each week. But certifying standards for these agencies don't really exist. They range from taking a 100-question quiz over the Internet to having to travel to a location to take in-depth written and practical exams. And there are a lot of *bad* certifications out there. However, there are also some very credible ones, the top, most

Check out the sites below to search for a trainer in your area. While you may not think you can afford a trainer, there are options, such as partner training and group training that can significantly lower the cost and make working with a fitness pro a reality—for both you and your pocketbook.

www.ideafit.com
www.acsm.org
www.acefitness.org
www.nsca-lift.org

respected being the American College of Sports Medicine (ACSM), the American Council on Exercise (ACE), and the

National Strength and Conditioning Association (NSCA). With that said, here are some top tips for choosing a personal trainer:

Check out their training. A certification from a credible association and/or an exercise-related college degree is a must. Not sure if a certification is credible? Ask for the organization's web site address, and check it out yourself. Their education sets the foundation for their knowledge. Also make sure they're furthering their education by taking continuing education courses.

Ask about their experience. How long have they been in the fitness field? What has their experience been? Do they specialize in any particular areas? Like anything else, the longer they've been doing it, the more experience they have to draw from.

Ask for personal references from past clients. Get several names and numbers of the trainer's previous and/or present clients and follow-up to see what kind of experience they've had with this trainer. Be sure to ask what, if any, relationship they have to the trainer. Relatives and good friends will, of course, be biased.

Interview the trainer. While the first meeting is for the trainer to meet you and see where you're at, it's also a time for you to interview him or her—remember, you're the one doing the hiring. Ask about the trainer's wellness philosophies, how much say you'll have in designing your program, and what *his/her* image of fitness is. These types of questions will help you determine if this trainer is a good fit with your own vision of fitness—and will help to increase your chances of success and a pleasurable experience.

Lifestyle and wellness coaching is fast entering the mainstream as a top profession to be in. And for good reason. Many feel that wellness and lifestyle coaching is going to bridge the gap between those who aren't living lives of wellness and the health and fitness industry. Coaching itself focuses on the client and her needs and desires. Rather than designing goals and a program for you, a coach works with you to help *you* determine and design your goals and your plan of action—much like what I've tried to do within the pages of this book. It is my hope that others in the fitness industry take note

> Sadly, fitness has become more about beauty than overall well-being. It's more about sex appeal than it is preventing disease. And it's more about creating the perfect body than it is being your best self. It's no wonder so many women haven't jumped onto the fitness bandwagon.

of the skills and techniques that coaches bring to our field, and adopt them to their own aspect of practice. It's a win-win situation.

Myths, Misnomers, and Misunderstandings

There are many myths surrounding fitness. Let's take a look at some and see if we can't clear up some of the muddied water.

You have to be athletic to be fit. I have a confession to make…I don't have natural athletic ability. It's funny, because I've fooled a lot of people into thinking I am naturally athletic, simply because I'm into fitness. And when I tell them that while I did play a couple of sports in high school, I was pretty horrible at them. Just ask my softball coach! How could I possibly have made the team? My high school was *very* small—try, 29-kids-small in my graduating class. They had to let everyone play, or they wouldn't have had a sports program! One thing you *must* realize is that fitness does not equate with athletic ability. You do not have to be a natural athlete—or even an unnatural athlete for that matter—to participate in fitness and to be fit. They are two separate things.

Exercise has to be done all at once to get any benefit from it. This is what we used to believe. But we now know that fitness can be broken up throughout the day, and you can still derive great benefits. Don't have a block of 30 minutes for your cardio? No problem! Can you do 10 minutes here, 10 minutes there, and another 10 minutes somewhere over there? Strength training can be broken up, too. Some push-ups before breakfast, crunches during coffee break, squats after lunch...the sky's the limit!

Low intensity, long duration exercise burns more fat. Again, it's what we thought at one point. LILD exercise used to be big in group fitness! Physiologically speaking, your body uses carbohydrates, which have been broken down into simple sugars, for its primary initial energy source. Some fat will be burned during this time, but sugar is the main source. Then after some time—15 or 20 minutes—the body starts switching over to more fat usage, as it begins to deplete the sugar source. So in order to burn more fat, you have to go beyond that first 20 minutes, hence, the 30-60 minute time frame. And this is still true—for lower intensity work. If you workout at a higher intensity, you will be burning more overall calories, including more fat calories. Because of this, you will burn as much fat in a shorter, higher intensity workout, as you do in a longer, lower intensity one.

Strength training will make you bulky. This is one of the biggest misconceptions between women and their dumbbells. We want long, lean, toned muscles—not big, bulky ones. Right? In order to build muscle, there are a couple of things you need: a stressed muscle, and testosterone (there are others, but these are two biggies). Now, I didn't say a stressed-out muscle. If that were the case, most of us wouldn't have to lift a finger! I said stressed muscles, which means the muscle must be placed under more work than it's used to. This is where lifting weights, using exercise bands, or even our own body weight comes in. These things all place added resistance on the muscle—beyond what it's used to.

The other thing you need is testosterone. Think you don't have any? Think again! It's not just for men! Women have testosterone in their bodies, too, just smaller quantities than men. The more testosterone you have, the easier it is to build muscle. The more muscle you have, the more your metabolism is revved up. Thus, the answer to the age-old question: why does *he* lose weight more quickly then I do? Men lose it faster, in large part, because they've got more muscle mass using up a greater number of calories. So back to our original question: can you get bulky from strength training? Sure! But chances are you won't. The female body builders you see gracing the pages of the hardcore magazines put in hours of training a day and follow very strict diets. They *want* to look that way (don't ask)! There's also a very good chance in this day and age that they're doing steroids (ever wonder why most of them look and sound more like men?).

You may appear a bit bulky as you first start growing muscle. But it's not the muscle that's making you bulky—it's the layer of fat over the muscle. As you continue to workout, that fat is going to gradually become less and less until one day you're going to be flexing in front of your mirror and realize, "Hey! I have a little muscle!"

But the benefits of strength training go way beyond just aesthetics. All that extra stress on the muscles is also going to the bones, which means they're getting stronger, and in turn, reducing your chance of osteoporosis. Being stronger as you get older also means you have less of a chance of falling. You can lead a more active life. And the literature also shows cardiovascular benefits from strength training. Most experts also agree that the best way to manage your waistline is through a combination of cardio, strength training, stress reduction, and eating well. After strength training for three or four weeks, you're going to notice a difference: your posture is going to improve, you're going to feel taller and stronger, and you're going to feel good about yourself!

Free weights are better than machines (or visa versa). When trying to decide which technique to use to strengthen your muscles, you're going to be faced with the option of using free weights or weight machines, especially if you join a club. Do a search on the Internet about which method is best, and all you're going to find is a bunch of opinions. Which one is "best" totally depends on you and which one you prefer—each has it's own pros and cons. Machines offer more safety, since you likely won't go beyond your range of motion. They can be good for strength training newbies, as there isn't much question about what you can or can't do on each machine. But with these safety nets come restrictions. Because each machine has restrictions regarding which muscles they work, they're not as functional, meaning, they don't necessarily work your muscles in the same ways they're used in every day life.

Free weights, on the other hand, offer much more freedom and functionality, but may be too aggressive for newcomers who haven't had proper instruction in them. They also tend to use more accessory muscles—helper muscles that work to stabilize the main working muscles—which means you're working more muscles at once (a good thing!). Another advantage of free weights is that they work your core—the muscles in the center of your body, including your abdominal muscles, back muscles, and pelvic floor muscles. This is because, unlike machines, which totally support your weight, the core muscles must work to support your weight while using the free weights. Free weights are also more economical and space efficient, as you can purchase a pair of dumbbells for a few bucks, do many exercises with them, and toss them under your bed when you're done, compared to the cost and space requirement of a home gym.

Of course, the options of what tools to use go beyond just free weights and machines. There are also exercise bands, exercise tubes, calisthenics…heck, you can use soup cans or milk jugs filled with sand or water if you want! Then there are the specialty-type disciplines, the two biggies being yoga and pilates. Not one of these options is any better than the other. It depends on what you prefer, what your goals are, and where you are on your journey in fitness.

You have to join a health club to really get fit. This is what the ads for health clubs would have you believe. I've also heard this come out of personal trainers' mouths. Again, this idea has to do with reserving fitness for a special class—in this case, for those who can afford the membership fees. But this is so far from the truth. You can get just as fit exercising at your own home or outside in the fresh air—it's simply another matter of preferences. For some, paying a membership fee to a club is a motivator to get them there to workout. They don't want to waste that money. For others, having to travel to go workout is de-motivating, as it takes too much time. I also know women who wouldn't step foot in a club with "all those beautiful women and gorgeous guys there." They're too embarrassed to go, because they feel they're too fat. Isn't this sad? The reason health clubs were started was so people could go to become healthier. And yet, those who need it most are too intimidated to go. If you think belonging to a health club would be motivating to you—if only you could find one that you dared go to—then I encourage you to look around. More and more "women only" clubs are popping up all over the place, and they're attracting women who normally would not step foot in another club.

You can pick and choose where you want the fat to disappear. Yeah. Sure—as long as you have a good plastic surgeon working along side you! That spot reducing myth is one of the oldest ones around. Moving one part of your body is not going to make the fat in that area move any faster, no matter how many leg lifts you do. Fat truly has a mind of its own! And it follows the old, "First hired, last fired" rule. As

212

any woman knows, the last-to-go is right where we want it to go first, usually in our "problem" areas.

With that said, there is such a thing as spot *training*. This simply means that you are training a specific area of the body, your abs or your saddlebag area, for instance. This does not mean you'll burn the fat from that area. It means that you're trying to tone that area and make it stronger. This leads us to the next myth...

Fat turns to muscle and muscle turns to fat. Not! This is yet another oldie that has captured our imaginations. These aren't stem cells, which can become whatever kind of cell we want them to. A muscle cell is a muscle cell, and a fat cell is a fat cell. One cannot become the other. You can lose fat and put on muscle or lose muscle and put on fat, but the two do not magically turn into each other.

You can't be fat and fit. Many of us fell for this one for a long time. But many "plus sized" men and women are shooting this theory to bits. There are some "off-the-weight-charts" women who can put many "fits-nice-and-neat-into-the-chart" women to shame. They have walked, biked, boogied, and lifted their way fit, just as anyone else can. They're just bigger.

You have to sweat buckets to get fit. One reason many of us avoid working out is because we don't want to have to change clothes to workout, take a shower, then change again...not to mention re-do our makeup, hair, jewelry, nails. I personally like to work up a good sweat at times, but not always. Some days, I don't want to mess with an extra shower and change of clothes. And research shows that I don't have to—and neither do you. Moderate exercise has many benefits, including reducing disease risk. So don't be afraid to strap on that pair of Rykas® walking shoes during your lunch break and take a nice, brisk, sweat-free walk!

Stepping Stones

- You must tailor fitness to you.
- Having a personal trainer or wellness coach work with you can be motivating.
- Make sure to carefully evaluate and interview potential personal trainers.
- There are many myths surrounding fitness—learn the truth!

CHAPTER SIXTEEN
Making
Fitness Fit You

O kay...now that I've totally berated the profession to which I belong—and will probably be excommunicated—let's discuss more of where *you* fit into the picture. Here are some more tools to toss into your toolbox, designed specifically for fitness.

Paint your self-portrait. Art students are often asked to paint self-portraits of themselves. This can be done literally, by looking into a mirror to create a mirror image of their physical selves, or it can be done more abstractly. The abstract reflects more of the artists' characters and what traits they feel they have. They might choose certain colors, shapes, or brush strokes to reflect this, or maybe an object. For instance, if one felt that she was strong and steady, she might choose a tall, straight pine tree to represent herself. Another one may choose an animal that reflects the same type of personality traits as she has. This same idea works with developing your own vision or self-image of fitness. In order to become successful with fitness and make it work for you, you need to be able to picture yourself fitting into fitness. The problem, as we've already discussed at some length, is that fitness has become prepackaged and pre-molded. In order for you to find success in fitness, you've had to squeeze yourself into that mold. This may work temporarily—like all the diets you've squeezed yourself into—but it doesn't work for the long haul. Instead, you need to create your own vision of fitness and how fitness fits *you*.

A Coaching Moment

Have the media images of fitness been stumbling blocks for you? Do you feel as though you've been trying to squeeze yourself into fitness...and you just can't seem to make it fit? If so, create your own image of fitness. What do *you* think fitness should look like? How do you envision yourself being fit? What do you look like? What do you wear? What activities do you do? Become like a tailor and create a fitness suit, tailor-made just for you. Also try putting another face to it. Look for role models in your own community—people who more closely match your own image—and use them, rather than the media, as your fitness role models. And don't be shy about letting them know you've chosen them as your role models. Letting them know they are an encouragement to you, will in turn, encourage them.

Believe that you belong. Fitness can come across as this sort of exclusive club, where only the already fit can belong. If you don't meet the minimum fitness requirements—body fat under

Fitness is for everyone, regardless of size, shape, or age. It's going to be women like you who change the face of fitness. I could talk until I'm blue in the face, but until *you* take action, and do something about it, 'the fit get fitter, and the fat get fatter' will continue to be the mantra of the day. Stop believing you're not 'fit to be fit,' and just start moving!

a certain percentage, participating in the "right" activities, wearing the "right" clothes, and just having the overall "right look"—you don't belong and you won't be allowed to join. Another part of changing your self-image is to believe that you *do* belong. While it would seem that there is some elusive fitness club, you need to change your perspective and hand yourself a membership card. Don't let the media images prevent you from joining this club. Know that fitness is for everyone—even you—and make it work for you.

A Coaching Moment

How do you feel about physical activity? Do you enjoy it? If not, what do you think may be the cause of your feelings? List the reasons why you don't enjoy exercise. You may have to go back in time to your childhood. What were your feelings toward P.E.? Were you always the last one chosen for the teams during recess? Did you feel awkward as a kid playing games, because you didn't have natural athletic ability? Journal out your feelings. Then go back and write down the ways exercise will make you feel good about yourself. Name the activities you would enjoy doing or trying now. Set a date to do one of them...and do it!

What's Your Attitude Like?

What has your attitude been about fitness in general? This is closely related to your fitness self-image, but rather than envisioning how you fit into the picture, concentrate instead on how you feel about fitness and moving your body. Does it make you happy? Feel good? Joyful? Do you have "glad-itude" when it comes to fitness...or "bad-itude?" Do you hate exercise? Dread the thought of having to do it? Because your fitness self-image and your attitude are so closely intertwined, the one can't help but affect the other. If you have felt like you don't belong in fitness, then chances are, your attitude about fitness isn't going to be too positive. But as your image of fitness changes, so will your attitude. And as your attitude becomes more positive, it will give you that old, "I can do this!" feeling. A positive attitude can go a long way in life, and get you further than you ever thought you could go—no matter what the challenge.

One thing that may help with your attitude toward exercise is to rename it. Yep. You heard right. Give exercise a new name! Here's your chance to change history, start a new trend. Believe it or not, exercise is nurturing to your body—unless you're abusing it, which is the other end of the spectrum from not exercising at all. But the words "exercise" and "workout" sound, well, so much like work! Come up with a name for exercise that sounds more nurturing—something you can relate to, that will make you feel good about doing it. Then, create a "be good to me basket," filled with fitness goodies—workout shoes, water bottle, hand weights or bands, favorite video, pedometer, etc. Another wonderful thing to do is wrap up little "Good for me!" gifts and keep them in your basket for those days when you need a little pat on the back. The gifts can be as simple as your favorite, inspiring quotes, little gift certificates to your favorite local shops or restaurants, or even a little chocolate inspiration! Even better, enlist your beau to do the gifts, or have a friend do them—then do the same for them.

Does Fitness Fit Your Personality?

This has more to do with the actual nitty-gritty of fitness than the image does. For example, studies show that morning exercisers tend to stick with it—get it over with in the morning and get on with your day. But you're not a morning person, and are lucky to make it out of bed with enough time to get everyone off in the morning. Here's another one: we tend to have this perception of fitness that only certain activities "count." If it doesn't fit within the walls of a health club, it's not as good. Guidelines for the "appropriate" exercises used to be quite strict. For instance, it used to be thought that the best—and only real way—to burn fat was through low intensity, long duration exercise. But what if you don't have that much time to put into working out, or if you prefer higher intensity, shorter duration work? Now we know that whether you choose to workout at a lower intensity and longer duration or a higher intensity and shorter duration, you'll gain benefits from either one.

When I wrote an article on fitness personalities I received some good feedback. One reader wrote in that she was so relieved to realize that there wasn't something wrong with the fact that she found morning exercise so repulsive. Her boyfriend had been dragging her out of bed in the morning to go running, because that's when it was supposed to be done. But she didn't feel like she was benefiting from it as much as she did when she went later in the day. You *do* have options when it comes to fitness! As I had written, no one plan fits everyone. We all have different personalities and preferences, and your fitness plan should be tailored to *you*. If you want to delve deeper into this topic, an excellent reference is *The*

Fitness Instinct by Peg Jordan (Rodale, 1999). In it, she gives a nice test for you to pinpoint your own fitness personality. You can also take a jab at the handy dandy quiz in the section below, if you'd like, or consider the "Coaching Moment" to get you thinking about your own movement style. If you haven't been nurturing your body with movement, designing your program with your personality and preferences in mind will increase the likelihood you'll stick with it. Once you've regained your sense of joy that evolves around moving your body (yes, you can feel good about moving your body!), don't be shy about venturing out of your specific movement style. Be adventurous! Try activities that don't necessarily fit your style, but that you think would be fun and would like to try.

A Coaching Moment

If you could do whatever you wanted for physical activity, what would it be? Fitness should be about you. Try to break out of the boxed-in-perceptions of what fitness should be. What activities did you enjoy when you were a child? Are any of them ones you could do now?

What's Your Movement Style?

Take this quick quiz to give yourself an idea of your movement style. This isn't meant, however, to lock you into one style. It's simply meant to be a tool you can use to help regain your joy of movement. By designing your fitness plan around your personality, you increase the likelihood of enjoying it and sticking with it.

1. I consider myself to be mostly an:
   a. extrovert
   b. introvert

2. My motivation comes mostly from:
   a. other people.
   b. within myself.

3. I would rather be:
   a. outside.
   b. inside.

4. I am a:
   a. morning person.
   b. night owl.

5. I believe:
   a. slow and steady wins the race.
   b. in going all out with all I've got.

6. I prefer to do projects in:
   a. small chunks of time.
   b. all at once, in one sitting.

Interpreting Your Results

Questions 1, 2, and 3: Chances are if you chose 'a' for number one, you probably also chose 'a' for numbers two and three. This just means that you're a people person, and get great pleasure from socializing. This also means that you'll probably get great benefits from working out in group settings. Whether it's yoga, kickboxing, or group strength training, sign on!

Because much of your motivation comes from others, it's also a good idea for you to workout with a buddy, especially if the classes aren't your thing. If you chose 'b' you probably have a strong individual personality, in which case most group classes aren't your style, with the exception of yoga and martial arts, which really focus on the individual. While a gym setting may seem suffocating, being outside frees your spirit. Choose home and outdoor activities for the bulk of your workout and if you have to go to the gym, try to go during "low-traffic" times.

Question 4: Because there are pros and cons regarding whatever time of day you workout, a good rule of thumb is to workout during the time of day you have the most energy. If this is impossible due to your schedule, try rearranging your schedule or choosing your next highest energy peak. You may also find that you can do your cardio workout on a little less energy, but need more energy to do your strength training routine, or visa versa. It's different for everyone.

Question 5: If you chose 'a' you probably prefer lower intensity, longer duration types of exercise. There is nothing wrong with this—you just need to pencil in a little more time for your workouts, and in the long run you're going to gain more benefits if it means you'll stick with it. If you chose 'b' then high intensity interval training is just what the trainer ordered—hit it hard, get it over with.

Question 6: Those of you who chose 'a' may enjoy breaking up your exercise time throughout the day—ten minutes on the treadmill here, a few push-ups there, some jumping jacks here, several crunches there... And those of you who preferred 'b,' the old fashioned, all at once method is probably better for you.

But I Just Don't Have Time!

This is probably the number one reason for not working out. Time! Or I should say, the lack of it. You're probably getting sick of hearing it, but go back and read the first two sections again if you still don't get this point. Most of us have too much "fluff" accumulating in our schedules that needs to be weeded out. One bump in the road you may run into is, what if the only available slot in your schedule, that could be used to workout, doesn't match your fitness personality? This is where not getting too overly attached to your personality comes in. You need to decide whether it will benefit you greater at this time to workout when you currently have a slot in your schedule, or whether you should try to rearrange your schedule to accommodate your personality. Which option is most likely to "stick?" Remember, too, that none of this is written in stone. It can always be changed.

A Coaching Moment

What excuses have you been using to avoid moving your body? Is lack of time one of them? Where could you squeeze in a few minutes of fitness? By starting with just a few minutes of exercise a day, you can get the feeling for it and gradually increase your time from there. This will also help you to see that it's not as intimidating as it might seem. You might even find yourself *enjoying* it! Being successful at a little bit of fitness is a catalyst for being successful at lifelong fitness.

Multitask

Combine fitness with other tasks. For example, park your car in a central location and walk to your errands. Are you early to a doctor's appointment (or are they running late)? Ask the receptionist how long the wait will be and use that time to take a quick walk. Read or listen to a book-on-tape while on the treadmill. Doing activities such as yoga or pilates can be a form of multitasking, because these types of activities work on several areas of fitness at once: cardio, strength, flexibility, balance, and stress relief.

Get out of your all-or-nothing mentality. Depending on your personality, you may be one of those types of people who think it has to be all or nothing—no matter what the "it" is. For instance, when I taught childbirth education classes, many women who wavered on the whole breastfeeding issue did so because they didn't want to be "tied down," or they wanted daddy or grandma to help partake in feeding the baby. I tried to show them that while exclusive breastfeeding is wonderful, you can combine both breast and bottle if that's more up your alley. It was a light bulb moment for many a mom-to-be, as they realized they had options—that some breastfeeding was better than none at all. And so it is with exercise. How many times have you looked at your watch and thought, "There's no sense in going for a walk now. I've only got ten minutes." That ten minutes is more than you've done right now—which is nothing. Take it and run (well, not literally run if you hate to run, but you know what I mean)! While we used to think that exercise had to be done all at once in order to gain any benefit, we now know it can be broken up throughout the day. And this is great for those of us who like to do things in smaller bites. It's also great for those of us who prefer to do it all at once, but are having a week (or two, or three...) when our schedules have taken over, not allowing us the time to get in longer workouts. It's all about options!

Stepping Stones

- Paint your own fitness self-portrait.
- Believe that you belong in fitness.
- Determine to become the new, true face of fitness.
- Determine to have "glad-itude" rather than "bad-itude" when it comes to fitness.
- Use your fitness personality as a guide when scheduling fitness into your life.
- Realize fitness isn't an all-or-nothing proposition.

CHAPTER SEVENTEEN

Design Your Own Personalized, "Indi-FIT-ual" Plan

While it certainly can be helpful to hire a trainer or coach to help you design a personalized fitness plan (what I like to call an "Indi-FIT-ual" plan—cute, huh?), it isn't necessary for everyone. By following a few key points, you can create a plan that fits you just right. Let's work step-by-step through the process of creating your own plan.

STEP ONE: **Determine what you are trying to accomplish.**
It's important to establish what you want to achieve before you actually set up any goals. In other words, what do you want the outcome to be to your fitness goals? Some possibilities are:

- fat loss
- increased muscular toning
- increased flexibility
- increased muscular strength and endurance
- increased cardiorespiratory strength and endurance
- decreased disease risk
- increased balance
- increased overall feelings of well-being
- decreased pain from a chronic injury

STEP TWO: Determine what you need to do to accomplish these outcomes. For example, if you desire to increase muscular strength and endurance, you'll need to start strength training. If you want to increase your cardiovascular strength and endurance, you'll have to add some cardio exercise. These are more straight-forward. Others aren't. For instance, if you want to increase your overall well-being, you'll have to decide what will help you with that. Strength training? Cardio exercise? Stress management? A combination of activities? Then there are the desires that everyone has an opinion about, namely, weight control. As we discussed previously, there are as many opinions on this topic as there are diets. You need to find what works for you, but chances are, it will involve some sort of equation of eating well, moving more, and managing your stress.

STEP THREE: Determine your motivation for these outcomes. Why do you want to achieve these end-results? What are the benefits of achieving these outcomes? Are these reasons powerful enough to motivate you to lasting success? Where are the motivations coming from? Are they coming from you, or from outside sources? Outside sources can include friends, family, your physician, that college reunion coming up in six months, the weight loss contest your company's wellness center is holding, this month's issue of *Exercise in the Buff* magazine… even the military, if you're planning on joining the Army! Write down your motivations to change, and decide if they're powerful enough to help you achieve your goals and make lasting, life-long changes

Sometimes, the toughest external motivation comes from our family. Your kids, husband, sisters, mother, second-cousin-once-removed all want you to lose weight, to exercise, to stop eating all those Krispy Kremes®. But if *you* don't have a real desire to do so, and you're doing it just to please them, there becomes a conflict of interest.

Sometimes, changing for someone else is enough motivation. But how healthy is it? Many times, the reason we're willing to change for others is out of fear—we're afraid of losing their love...and can *that* be healthy?

A Coaching Moment

Think waaaay back to the beginning chapters of this book when we discussed comparing ourselves to other women. Are you still using someone else's weight, size, or body appearance as your motivation to change? If so, do you think this is powerful enough to spur you on to achieve your goals? This type of external desire is not usually a lasting motivation, and just leads to disappointment. There will always be another body you'd rather have. Instead, try to focus on what you've got and how you can accomplish being the best "you," you can be.

STEP FOUR: **Write down your goals.** If you've forgotten the basics of goal writing, refer back to Chapter Eleven for a refresher. Start with your long-term goals. I recommend setting three-month goals as long-term goals. This is long enough for you to get something accomplished, but not so long it seems as though the time will never come. Once your three-month goals are set, break them down. Begin with the next week. What do you think you can accomplish in relation to your three-month goals in the next week? As an example: if one of your three-month goals is to consistently do a cardio workout five times a week, what would be a reasonable goal for the next week that would create a stepping stone toward this goal? Remember that all your goals should be SMART goals: short and specific; measurable (where possible); action-based; realistic, and time-specific.

STEP FIVE: **Set your plan in place.** Part of getting the ball rolling, is putting all this into writing—and then placing your plan where you'll see it daily. Hang your goals up some place obvious, where you can't ignore them. Also put into writing *how* you're going to get these goals done in the next week. Let's say that you want to go for two, 30-minute walks this week. That's a great goal! And it looks good on paper. But now you need to figure out a way to actually put your goal into action. Pencil it into your schedule. If your schedule is very unforgiving and isn't allowing time for this, how can you fit it in? Do you need to do it in chunks? Can you break down each walk into two 15-minute mini-walks? How about three 10-minute walks? Or is there something in your schedule that can be weeded out this week? Are there activities that can be consolidated? Can you combine your walk with something else? For instance, can you park your car and walk while doing errands?

A Coaching Moment

Consider your schedule for a moment. Are there activities that can be weeded out this week that will give you the time you need to reach your goals? What activities can be consolidated? Are you running errands every day? Can they be done on one day? Are you running to the store every day either because you forgot something or because you haven't

229

planned any further ahead for meals than the night before? What are some things you can do to become more efficient with your time?

STEP SIX: Prepare ahead for obstacles. Obstacles will happen, even with the best of intentions. So plan for them now. Write down potential hurdles you're likely to have to jump at some point. Then include possible solutions to these hurdles. As an example, let's go back to your walking goal of two 30-minute walks a week. And let's say that you've chosen to do this during your lunch hour. What might get in the way of you accomplishing this? Lunch-time parties? Meetings? Lunch outings? Temptation to work through lunch? Forgetting your walking shoes? Now write down some possible solutions to these setbacks. If you've set Monday and Wednesday as your walking days, and you know ahead of time about any parties, meetings, or outings, can you switch your walking days to different days that week? If you know you'll have trouble remembering to bring your walking shoes from home, can you have a pair to keep at work? What about that temptation to work through lunch? This is a toughie. And it brings me to my next point...

STEP SEVEN: Multitask. Multitasking can be a big time-saver. And there are several ways to combine tasks into one. For instance, we've already talked about walking while running errands. What about reading or watching the news while on your treadmill or exercise bike? While I was in the breastfeeding stage of my life (times four), I gave new meaning to the word multitask, as I could nurse while riding a stationary bike. I guess I was also working my upper body, too, as holding that baby up had to be working my muscles! You can also combine different components of fitness into one workout. Circuit training—alternating cardio, strength, and flexibility exercises—is a great way to do this. Disciplines such as yoga or pilates work on strength, cardio, flexibility, balance, and stress relief. Taking your kids or husband for a walk can be a great way to discuss your day and get some exercise in, too.

A couple of cautions on multitasking: first, you can multi-task so much that you are never focusing on one thing at a time. In doing so, you miss out on experiencing any pure joy associated with that activity. Second, you can be so into multitasking that you end up ignoring someone in need. For instance, let's say that you're folding laundry, reading the paper, making out your shopping list, and helping your daughter with her homework...all while chopping the veggies for supper and packing the next day's lunches. Who's missing out here? Both you and your daughter. Don't let your need to multitask due to an over-crowded schedule take the place of giving someone your undivided attention and love.

STEP EIGHT: Be accountable to someone. If you think about it, we're accountable to many different people in our lives, for many different things. We're accountable to our husbands. We're accountable to our bosses. We're even accountable to our children. And it also all works in reverse. Being accountable to someone helps keep us on our toes, and we're much more likely to get done what we need to do. This is a great concept when it comes to making changes and establishing new habits. Choose someone who will be firm and accept no excuses, but who is also warm, understanding, and nonjudgmental...and won't be sabotaging your efforts by offering excuses for you (there's nothing worse than having a saboteur as your accountability person!). This person should know your goals and what you expect to accomplish each week. And they should "check up" on you often to see how you're doing. Just knowing that you have to "report" to someone who isn't going to accept your excuses can be motivation enough to keep on track! It also helps to have someone you can bounce your goals off of, to get their opinion (are they reasonable?). Even better than one accountability partner is having several. This way, if one gets sidetracked or pulled away for whatever reason, you've got at least one other person to step in.

STEP NINE: **Revisit your goals each week.** It's important to take an honest look at what you've accomplished each week. Did you get your two walks in? If not, why? While this can be a painful process, it's necessary to honestly evaluate where you are and whether or not you're headed in the right direction. You're going to have setbacks. Take them, embrace them, learn from them. If you didn't accomplish your goals, what happened? What could you have done differently? Write it down. It's one thing to think it. It's another thing to see it written in your own handwriting. It personalizes it more and makes you own it—excuses and all!

STEP TEN: **Re-evaluate your three-month goals.** Also take time every few weeks to re-evaluate your three-month goals. Do they still follow the SMART principles? Were you over-enthusiastic (and unrealistic) when you originally chose these goals? Are you on track to meeting them? Have you already met them? Maybe you didn't give yourself enough credit and set goals that didn't stretch you enough. Three-month goals aren't written in stone. Revisit them once in a while and re-work them if necessary.

A Women in Wellness™ Success Story

To illustrate the importance of setting small, reachable, progressive goals, I'd like to introduce you to one of my clients, MaryAnn. One of MaryAnn's desires was to be able to play and keep up with her grandchildren. This was difficult for her to do carrying an extra 150 pounds. Because MaryAnn hadn't been active and had a desk job, we knew her fitness goals needed to start out small so that she could have success with them and gradually progress up to larger goals. MaryAnn and I set her first week's cardio goal at five minutes. Yep! Just five minutes, twice that week! Sound ridiculously small, you say? Well, for MaryAnn, it was just right. She was able to meet that goal—and all her other small stepping stones—and within three months had worked her fitness goals up to "30 minutes of cardio, five times a week" and "two strength training sessions a week." She now does interval training, adding spurts of higher intensity walking into her workout to further increase her cardiovascular capabilities.

MaryAnn also needed to rearrange her eating habits. She would go all day long without eating, and come home and binge. She now eats three meals and two to three snacks every day—and doesn't binge. She doesn't need to, because she's not putting her body into starvation mode. She has the occasional emotional eating setback, but she now recognizes what sets it off, and has a plan in place when she feels the draw to the refrigerator.

MaryAnn also doesn't focus on her weight. This is a new way of thinking for her, since with every diet she tried—and believe me, she's tried them all—weight was the focus. And while weight loss is certainly a fringe benefit, she now uses how her clothes fit, fitness progression, and her overall feeling of well-being as her assessment tools. MaryAnn—you are a Women in Wellness™ star!

Stepping Stones

- Determine what outcomes you want to accomplish with your fitness program, whether or not they are reasonable for you, and what you have to do to accomplish them.
- Figure out your motivations for what you want to accomplish, and whether or not they are strong enough to push you ahead.
- Keep track of your goals and plan and prepare for obstacles.
- Find at least one person to be accountable to.

AFTERWORD

Life's a Journey...do you know where your keys are?

hew! You made it through the book! Thanks for sticking with me! Before you run off to continue your journey, let's use this "rest area" to quickly retrace our steps so far:

The Landfill: It's really difficult to move forward in your journey if you refuse to dump your old baggage. For many of us, this is simply a choice. Others may require more intensive work. I encourage you to seek professional counseling. Sometimes you must move backward in order to ultimately move forward. If you choose, instead, to lug all that baggage with you, be prepared for delays—loooong delays!

Attitude Check: You can't control how others will act—but you can control your reaction to them! Deal openly and honestly with your healthy living saboteurs, and make decisions based on optimal thinking, rather than unbalanced— too positive or too negative—decision-making.

Bridges: Remember *desire*, *choose*, *plan*, and *action*? These are the bridges to close the gap between old habits and creating new ones. While there will be times you will be able to skip one or more of the steps, they are normally all necessary for success.

Vision: How do you get somewhere if you don't know where you're headed? You don't! You must have a vision of where you want to be—then check it for the three R's: making sure it's realistic, reachable, and reasonable. Stretch yourself—but not so far that it's not possible to live out your vision!

Live Your Life on Purpose, Not by Accident: By living your life according to your reason for being here, you stop busy living, and start passionate living. No more time excuse!

Goals: Without goals, you live life floundering around, wandering from one event to the next. By combining purposeful living and setting your goals according to that purpose, you greatly increase your productivity and efficiency—not to mention your fulfillment.

Reflect: There is a constant reassessment process that needs to go on in order to make sure you are setting appropriate goals. Are the goals being set according to your needs and purpose— or someone else's? Is it really a mold in disguise, intended for someone else? If so, readjust the goal according to what you need—and break the mold!

While this is the last paragraph of the last chapter of this book, it is my hope and prayer that this is just the beginning for you. Yeah, that's right—I'm praying for *you*! I'm praying for each and every one of you who takes the time to read this book and desires to make healthy changes. I'd love to know how you're doing in your journey in wellness—and I'm only a click away! Drop me a line at carrie@womeninwellness.com, or at Champion Press, 4308 Blueberry Road, Fredonia, WI 53021.

I may use your story to help inspire other women to wellness—and that would fulfill one of the reasons we're doing this in the first place—to take better care of ourselves, so that we can give in more meaningful ways. Here's to *your* wellness!

Good Reads

On Food and Eating

Intuitive Eating: A Revolutionary Program that Works by Evelyn Tribole, M.S., R.D., and Elyse Resch, M.S., R.D.

Un-Dieting: Un-Doing the Diet Mentality...and Staying Fit Forever! by Jackie Jaye-Brandt, M.A., MFT with Diana Lipson-Burge, R.D.

When You Eat at the Refrigerator, Pull Up a Chair: 50 Ways to Feel Thin, Gorgeous, and Happy (When You Feel Anything But) by Geneen Roth

The Rush Hour Cook Series by Brook Noel.
> *The Rush Hour Cook's Presto Pasta*
> *The Rush Hour Cook's One-Pot Wonders*
> *The Rush Hour Cook's Family Favorites*
> *The Rush Hour Cooks Effortless Entertaining*

The Rush Hour Cook's Weekly Wonders by Brook Noel

Saving Diner: The Menus, Recipes, and Shopping Lists to Bring your Family Back to the Table by Leanne Ely, CNC.

Mayo Clinic on Healthy Weight: Answers to Help You Achieve and Maintain the Weight That's Right for You put out by the Mayo Clinic

On Living Life on Purpose/Finding Meaning

You Can Experience a Purposeful Life by James Emery White

The Purpose Driven Life: What on Earth Am I Here For? by Rick Warren

Passion on Purpose: Discovering and Pursuing a Life that Matters by Dr. Deborah Newman

On Body Image
Loving Your Body: Embracing Your True Beauty in Christ by Dr. Deborah Newman

On Self-Worth/Self-Esteem
A Woman's Search for Worth: Finding Fulfillment as the Woman God Intended You to Be by Dr. Deborah Newman

The New Hide or Seek: Building Self-Esteem in Your Child by Dr. James Dobson

On Fitness/Your Body
Fit From Within: 101 Simple Secrets to Change Your Body and Your Life—Starting Today and Lasting Forever by Victoria Moran

The Fitness Instinct: The Revolutionary New Approach to Healthy Exercise That is Fun, Natural, and No Sweat by Peg Jordan

On Self-Nurturing
365 Simple Pleasures: Daily Suggestions for Comfort and Joy collected by Susannah Seton

Self-Nurture: Learning to Care for Yourself as Effectively as You Care for Everyone Else by Alice D. Domar, Ph.D.

On Organization/De-Cluttering
Let Go of Clutter by Harriet Schechter

Stop Clutter from Stealing Your Life: Discover Why You Clutter and How You Can Stop by Mike Nelson

Home Management 101: A Guide for Busy Parents by Debbie Williams

A Simple Choice: A Practical Guide for Saving Your Time, Money, and Sanity by Deborah Taylor-Hough

Sink Reflections by Marla Cilley

Sidetracked Home Executives: From Pigpen to Paradise by Pam Young and Peggy Jones

On Changing Your Habits
Mind Over Matter: Personal Choices for a Lifetime of Fitness by Susan Cantwell. Download the e-book at www.lifestylecoaching.ca.

On Changing Your Mind
Optimal Thinking: How to Be Your Best Self by Rosalene Glickman, Ph.D.

The Mass Market Woman: Defining Yourself as a Person in a World That Defines You By Your Appearance by Linda McBryde, M.D.

More Cool Tools
The MIO™ heart rate monitor and lifestyle watch is a tool I use to help gauge the intensity of my workouts. The greatest thing about this little device is that there is no chest strap. If you're familiar with other heart rate monitors, they require a strap that connects around your chest—not always the most comfortable thing for women! And it doubles as a watch, too,

so you get more bang for your buck. You can buy a MIO™ at your local sports shop, or check them out at www.gophysical.com.

The DIGI-WALKER™ pedometer is a great thing to use to gauge your distance while walking or running. It can also be used to see how many steps a day you take and help you determine if you're active enough. Did you know that there are health benefits to taking at least 10,000 steps a day—the equivalent of walking about five miles? By doing so, you will burn between 2,000 to 3,500 extra calories a week (assuming you aren't all ready walking that much). However, if you're one that tends to get stuck on numbers—and goes into a major depression when you don't meet your number goal—you may want to wait on this one. Look for DIGI-WALKERS™ at your local sports shop or log onto www.new-lifestyles.com.

A stability ball is something nearly all women should have in their toolbox. They are so versatile and allow you to do many more exercises than you could normally do without one. They're especially great for core work. You can find stability balls at your local department store, sports shop, and many online stores, such as www.bodytrends.com.

The Diet Plate®, as I mentioned before, has a bad name, but is a really great tool for those of you who need some practical guidance with portion sizes. They offer separate plates for men, women, and children, and there's also a bowl for those food items that would have a difficult time staying on the plate! Check them out at www.thedietplate.com.

BIBLIOGRAPHY

Chapter 1

You Are Special (Crossway Books, 1997) Max Lucado

Chapter 2

The Body Burden: Living in the Shadow of Barbie (Blue Note Publications, 2000) Stacey Handler

"Behind Closed Doors" with Joan Lunden (LMNO Productions, as seen on A&E Channel)

The Mass Market Woman: Defining Yourself as a Person in a World that Defines You by Your Appearance (Crowded Hour Press, 1999) Linda McBryde, M.D.

Chapters 3 and 4

When Food is Love: Exploring the Relationship Between Eating and Intimacy (Plume, 1992) Geneen Roth

Chapter 6

Making Aromatherapy Creams and Lotions (Storey Books, 2000) Donna Maria

Chapter 8

Sidetracked Home Executives: From Pigpen to Paradise (Warner Books, 2001) Pam Young, Peggy Jones

Chapter 10

Optimal Thinking: How to be Your Best Self (Wiley, 2002)
Rosalene Glickman, Ph.D.

Mind Over Matter: Personal Choices for a Lifetime of Fitness
(Stoddart, 1999) Susan Cantwell

Chapter 11

*Passion on Purpose: Discovering and Pursuing a Life that
Matters Most* (Tyndale House Publishers, 2003) Deborah
Newman, Ph.D.

Chapter 16

*The Fitness Instinct: The Revolutionary New Approach to
Healthy Exercise that is Fun, Natural, and No Sweat,* (Rodale
Press, 1999) Peg Jordan

About
Carrie Myers Smith...

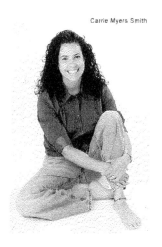

Carrie Myers Smith

Carrie Myers Smith has a bachelor's degree in exercise science and health education and is a trained Wellcoaches™ wellness coach. She's also the co-founder and president of Women in Wellness™ and a contributing editor and columnist for *Energy for Women* magazine.

You may contact Carrie by writing to:

Carrie Myers Smith
c/o Champion Press, Ltd.
4308 Blueberry Road
Fredonia WI 53021

Checkout these online services brought to you by Champion Press, Ltd.

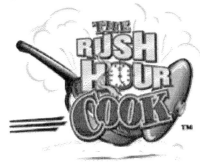

WWW.RUSHHOURCOOK.COM

Quick recipes.
Fun trivia.
Real advice.
Join the free "Daily Rush" cooking club.

THE FIVE RULES OF RUSH HOUR RECIPES:

1. All ingredients may be pronounced accurately through the phonetic use of the English Language.

2. Each ingredient can be located in the market without engaging on a full-scale scavenger hunt.

3. No list of ingredients shall be longer than the instructions.

4. Each recipe is durable enough to survive the Queen-of-Incapable Cooking and elicit a compliment.

5. The Rush Hour Cook's finicky child will eat it—or some portion of it.

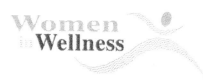

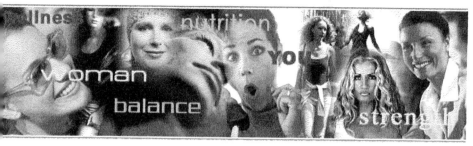

www.womeninwellness.com

IT'S ALL ABOUT YOU!
fitness...with a twist

What's different about Women in Wellness?

1. A whole-approach to wellness, covering physical, emotional and spiritual health
2. Interactive one-on-one coaching and customized planning
3. Sister in Success support program
4. We give you points, redeemable for prizes as you reach your goals!

change your life with a click...
FREE ONLINE WELLNESS CLUB!

Also available
from Champion Press, Ltd.

by Brook Noel a.k.a. The Rush Hour Cook
The Rush Hour Cook: Family Favorites by Brook Noel $5.95

The Rush Hour Cook: One-Pot Wonders by Brook Noel $5.95

The Rush Hour Cook: Effortless Entertaining by Brook Noel $5.95

The Rush Hour Cook: Presto Pasta by Brook Noel $5.95

The Rush Hour Cook: Weekly Wonders $16

by Deborah Taylor-Hough
Frozen Assets: Cook for a Day, Eat for a Month $14.95
Frozen Assets Lite & Easy: Cook for a Day, Eat for a Month $14.95
Frozen Assets Reader Favorites: Cook for a Day, Eat for a Month $25
Mix and Match Recipes: Creative Recipes for Busy Kitchens $9.95
A Simple Choice: A Practical Guide to Saving Your Time, Money and Sanity $14.95

Also available:
365 Quick, Easy and Inexpensive Dinner Menus by Penny E. Stone
(Over 1000 recipes!)

The Frantic Family Cookbook: mostly healthy meals in minutes by Leanne Ely $29.95 hardcover, $14.95 paperback

Healthy Foods: an irreverent guide to understanding nutrition and feeding your family well by Leanne Ely $19.95

The Complete Crockery Cookbook: create spectacular meals with your slow cooker by Wendy Louise $16

Crazy About Crockery: 101 Easy & Inexpensive Recipes for Less than .75 cents a serving by Penny Stone

TO ORDER
read excerpts, sample recipes, order books and more at
www.championpress.com
or send a check payable to Champion Press, Ltd. to 4308 Blueberry Road, Fredonia, WI 53021. Please include $3.95 shipping & handling for the first item and $1 for each additional item.

Also available
from Champion Press, Ltd.

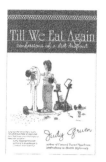

Till We Eat Again: Confessions of a Diet Dropout
will be loved by any and all who have attempted to
lose weight. Author Judy Gruen tries everything from
belly dancing to boot camp, in her attempt to shed
pounds before a high school reunion. Treat yourself to
a laugh!

**Healthy Foods: an irreverant guide to
understanding nutrition and feeding your
family well...** Tired of health food that tastes
weirder than It looks? Let Leanne Ely change
your diet with this part cookbook part nutrition
guide. You'll find that not only can healthy
eating taste great—it can be easy and enjoyed by
kids, too!

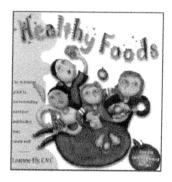

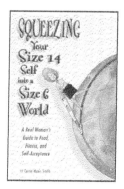

Squeezing Your Size 14 Self into a Size Six World
Weight loss—diets—it's the modern day nemesis of
most every woman. Plagued with unrealistic
expectations, poor body image and an unsuccessful
dieting track record, women are still hunting for the
"cure" to get the shape they desire. Carrie Myers
Smith, a contributing editor of *Energy* Magazine, has
been there and learned that life isn't about counting
calories or pounds but about a total wellness program
that addresses internal and external needs of a whole
life. Also available a companion workbook and
journal.